Empowered Patients, Empowered Care: Partnering for Healthier You

Fedor

First Printing, 2024

Table of Contents

Chapter 1 - Introduction

"If we do not engage consumers, patients and family members in health care processes, we will not be effective at eliminating inequalities and improving health for all."

– Kalahan Taylor-Clark (2012 April 12)

While not new concepts, patient-centred care and measurement are important in determining how well health care is delivered and how responsive the system is to patients' wants and needs (Larson, Sharma, Bohren, & Tunçalp, 2019). Ensuring health care that patients receive is in alignment with their wishes has been determined to not only improve outcomes, but have patients more engaged and involved in their care (Larson et al., 2019). With the publishing of the Institute for Healthcare Improvement's triple aim[1], the incorporation of patient-centred care has become a fundamental tenet in health care delivery (Institute of Medicine, 2001; Larson et al., 2019). By ensuring care is patient-centred, which is loosely defined as care that considers a patient's wants, needs and values, there is general agreement in the literature that there are both cost savings and outcome improvement as patients share responsibility for their care (Institute of Medicine, 2001). Unfortunately, determining how much a system is patient-centred remains problematic as it is a multi-dimensional concept that involves patients, the health care team, health organizations and health systems at large. While broad metrics on patient-centred care are difficult to ascertain, research and practice have demonstrated that patient experience, when combined with other outcomes data, can help determine how centred patient care is (Canadian Institute for Health Information [CIHI], 2017; Beattie, Murphy, Atherton, & Lauder, 2015; Chiu et al., 2014).

[1] Triple Aim refers to improving the patient experience of care, improve the health of populations and reducing the per capita cost of care. See Institute of Medicine (2001) for additional information

Patient Experience

Although there is a large body of literature on patient experience, there has not been agreement on a definition (Wolf, Niederhauser, Marshburn, & LaVela, 2014). Lack of a standard definition has not stopped jurisdictions worldwide from incorporating patient experience as part of measuring and improving health system performance (Canadian Institute for Health Information [CIHI], 2017; Sitzia & Wood, 1997). For this book, patient experience is defined as "the sum of all interactions shaped by an organization's culture, that influence patient perceptions across the continuum of care." (The Beryl Institute, n.d.)

Measures of patient experience are used to determine if an event designed to improve a patient's experience occurred. For example, a measure may ask if patients felt their values and needs were considered when conversing with health care professionals. Patients who have their values considered are more likely to follow their health care professionals' advice, leading to improvements in health outcomes (Fors, Taft, Ulin, & Ekman, 2016). While there are positive benefits to ensuring care is patient-centred, there are also unintended consequences of its measurement. The same improvement in relationships with health care professionals could coax health care providers to prescribe medications that a patient requests instead of medications that improve outcomes as an attempt to receive higher feedback scores (Zgierska, Rabago, & Miller, 2014). While scores can be manipulated, as long as an instrument is reliable and has high internal validity, the data gained should still be considered valid (Beattie et al., 2015).

The Hospital Consumer Assessment of Healthcare Providers and Systems (HCAHPS) was the first national standardized patient experience survey in the United States of America (Centers for Medicare and Medicaid Services [CMS], 2017). It has become a standard of measurement and is used to penalize and reward hospitals for performance (Mehta, 2015). An unintended consequence is that health care administrators may only focus on improving their HCAHPS scores without examining experiences that have meaning for patients. Ranard et al. (2016) determined that while the HCAHPS is a necessary longitudinal survey, the HCAHPS was missing experiences that patients found important. Without focusing on these other areas of concern, their conclusion was it would be difficult to improve health care as a whole.

Research Context

In 2016, Ranard et al. evaluated the use of online social media reviews as an adjunct source of information to the HCAHPS. The reviews were categorized using natural language processing, which used computers to classify the data and then humans interpreted the results. Ranard's team identified many positive benefits of utilizing social media reviews to supplement traditional survey methods. Social media reviews are freely available, are continuously updated and often link the experience of an event and a specific outcome (Hawkins, DeLao, & Hung, 2016). In addition to capturing data relevant to traditional surveys, they also captured patients' voices, specifically what mattered most. From a technological perspective, this data capture and analysis also benefited through its use of natural language processing, as they processed hundreds of thousands of reviews and gained contextually accurate information without reading each review. Ranard et al. (2016) concluded that not only were social media reviews a viable supplement to traditional patient experience surveys, they also provided information on issues not captured by the HCAHPS.

In 2013, the Canadian Institute for Health Information (CIHI) released a measurement framework to measure the performance of the Canadian health care system (Canadian Institute for Health Information [CIHI], 2013). CIHI's Health System Performance Measurement Framework unified health system performance and population health measurement. Part of this framework was the inclusion of patient experience to measure patient-centred care. However, the framework was designed to compare the system's different levels and did not include individual or population-based needs and wants (Canadian Institute for Health Information [CIHI], 2015). CIHI released the Canadian Patient Experience Survey – Inpatient Care (CPES-IC) in 2014. It is a survey tool based on HCAHPS but adds questions specific to the Canadian health care system (Canadian Institute for Health Information [CIHI], 2014). Additional information about the CPES-IC can be found in Chapter 2. Currently, the survey is available for jurisdictions across Canada to submit their data; however, as of June 2021, only six provinces were submitting data (Canadian Institute for Health Information [CIHI], 2021). Although survey participation rates amongst provinces are not high, the available data can still provide the opportunity to draw conclusions about patients' experience in the Canadian healthcare system. However, it is possible the CPES-IC, like the HCAHPS, may not be as helpful to Canadian policymakers and health organizations in detecting what concerns Canadian patients and their families.

With the addition of the CPES-IC as Canada's national patient experience survey, it is of interest to determine if the results of Ranard et al. (2016) hold in the Canadian context. In particular, do social media reviews contain relevant information to policy makers and patients? Can these reviews provide administrators and healthcare professionals with information to improve their patients' care? Given that little research of this nature has been published in Canadian health care literature, it is of interest to explore how these tools can potentially aid nursing and health care at large. Although there are many potential avenues of exploration when using patient experience, the promise of using natural language processing to capture and process data quickly is of interest. When processes are made efficient and cost-effective, there may be additional benefits. This work will focus on answering questions similar to Ranard et al. (2016), as it is undetermined if the results will hold when using the CPES-IC. This work is exploratory, and the focus will be on determining proof of concept.

Research Questions

Given this research's context, this thesis's primary purpose is to determine if the results of Ranard et al. (2016) hold true in the Canadian context; therefore, the research questions are:

1) Do Google free-text user reviews of hospitals in British Columbia contain information captured in domains of the Canadian Patient Experience Survey – Inpatient Care?
2) Do these same free-text user reviews also contain information not captured in the domains of the Canadian Patient Experience Survey – Inpatient Care?

Chapter 2 – Review of Relevant Literature

Introduction

Before delving into the research, it is helpful to understand the concepts of patient-centred care, patient experience, patient satisfaction, and how these concepts are related. Following will be a review of the literature on measuring patient experience and discussing possible gaps.

Patient-Centred Care

Patients that receive patient-centred care have demonstrated improvement in their health outcomes (Rathert, Williams, McCaughey, & Ishqaidef, 2015). There is also evidence to suggest that patient-centred care improves health care utilization and efficiency (Larson et al., 2019). It becomes essential to ensure that patients are receiving care that is patient-centred.

The Institute of Medicine (IOM) [2001] defines the concept of Patient-Centred Care as "providing care that is respectful of, and responsive to, individual patient preferences, needs and values, and ensuring that patient values guide all clinical decisions" pg.6. The IOM paraphrased from the Picker Institute that defines Patient-Centred Care as care organized around the patient (Frampton et al., 2008). Although a simple definition, Genteis, Edgman-Levitan, Daley, & Delbanco (1993) explain, there are eight dimensions that encompass Patient-Centred Care. These include:

1. Respect for patients' values, preferences and expressed needs
2. Coordination and integration of care
3. Information, communication and education
4. Physical comfort
5. Emotional support and alleviation of fear and anxiety

6. Involvement of family and friends
7. Continuity and transition
8. Access to care

According to the Picker Institute, being mindful of these eight dimensions when providing patient care ensures that care is patient-centred.

A growing body of evidence indicates that being inclusive of these eight dimensions does improve patient outcomes (Brännström & Boman, 2014; Goldfarb, Bibas, Bartlett, Jones, & Khan, 2017; Vincent et al., 2016). However, measuring patient-centred care is difficult as the dimensions are influenced by organizational culture, staff culture, and a patient's background and previous health care experiences (Fix et al., 2018). There is not yet agreement in the literature on quality indicators to measure patient-centred care, making it difficult to determine how effective interventions or improvements affect patient care (Santana et al., 2019). Patient-centred care is often used interchangeably with patient experience; however, they are distinct concepts. The assessment of patient experience is often used to measure patient-centred care (Larson et al., 2019).

Patient Experience

Measurement of patients' experiences has also been compared to measuring patient satisfaction (Cleary, 2016). According to Larson et al. (2019), patient satisfaction is considered an outcome of the care experience. Cleary (2016) has shown that satisfaction is often limited to meeting patient expectations which are seen as subjective measures. He describes patient satisfaction where patients can be satisfied with care that is not high quality and can also be dissatisfied with care that is considered high quality (Cleary, 2016; Larson et al., 2019). Whereas determining what events occurred for a patient from a patient's perspective is objective

(Cleary (2016); Drain & Clark (2004); and Lord & Gale (2014)). For example, the HCAHPS asks, "how often did nurses treat you with courtesy and respect (CMS, 2020)"? Being treated with courtesy and respect is a fundamental right when receiving healthcare and ensures trust between health care workers and patients (Larson et al., 2019).

Determining the patient's experiences removes the dynamics between a patient's perception of their health and the perception of care delivered. Instead of focusing on subjective feelings, patient experience surveys focus on determining what events did or did not occur during a health care encounter as this has been discussed as a way to assess if specific experiences improved patient outcomes (Cleary, 2016; Drain & Clark, 2004; Lord & Gale, 2014). The development of patient experience surveys by the Picker Institute culminated in the creation of the Consumer Assessment of Health Care Providers and Systems (CAHPS) survey. The CAHPS is considered a gold standard patient experience survey that measures quality of health care delivery through patient experience measurement (Cleary, 2016). Survey questions are focused on the occurrence of evidence-based events that have demonstrated improvement in health outcomes. The CAHPS survey assesses a patient's experiences related to the Picker eight dimensions (Edgman-Levitan & Cleary, 1996). Although there is little literature directly comparing the Picker dimensions with the CAHPS domains, it has been suggested that the Picker dimensions were the basis for the CAHPS questions (Newswire, 2003). In Table 2.1, I have mapped the eight Picker dimensions to the March 2020 Hospital CAHPS (HCAHPS) survey. The HCAHPS consists of twenty-nine items, including nineteen items that assess ten domains of concern, three items that screen for additional questions, and seven items for demographic purposes (Centers for Medicare and Medicaid Services [CMS], n.d.). I excluded the demographic and screening questions as these do not assess a patient's hospital experience. For a full copy of the HCAHPS survey please see Appendix A.

HCAHPS Domain	HCAHPS Question	Picker Dimension(s)
Nurse communication	During this hospital stay, how often did nurses treat you with courtesy and respect?	• Respect for patients' values, preferences and expressed needs • Emotional support and alleviation of fear and anxiety • Information, communication and education
	During this hospital stay, how often did nurses listen carefully to you?	• Respect for patients' values, preferences and expressed needs • Emotional support and alleviation of fear and anxiety • Information, communication and education
	During this hospital stay, how often did nurses explain things in a way you could understand?	• Respect for patients' values, preferences and expressed needs • Emotional support and alleviation of fear and anxiety • Information, communication and education
Responsiveness of hospital staff	During this hospital stay, after you pressed the call button, how often did you get help as soon as you wanted it?	• Respect for patients' values, preferences and expressed needs • Emotional support and alleviation of fear and anxiety • Physical comfort • Access to care
Doctor communication	During this hospital stay, how often did doctors treat you with courtesy and respect?	• Respect for patients' values, preferences and expressed needs • Emotional support and alleviation of fear and anxiety • Information, communication and education
	During this hospital stay, how often did doctors listen carefully to you?	• Respect for patients' values, preferences and expressed needs • Emotional support and alleviation of fear and anxiety • Information, communication and education

	During this hospital stay, how often did doctors explain things in a way you could understand?	• Respect for patients' values, preferences and expressed needs • Emotional support and alleviation of fear and anxiety • Information, communication and education
Cleanliness of hospital environment	During this hospital stay, how often were your room and bathroom kept clean?	• Physical comfort
Quietness of hospital environment	During this hospital stay, how often was the area around your room quiet at night?	• Physical comfort
Responsiveness of hospital staff	How often did you get help in getting to the bathroom or using a bedpan as soon as you wanted?	• Physical comfort • Access to care
Communication about medicines	Before giving you any new medicine, how often did hospital staff tell you what the medicine was for?	• Information, communication and education
	Before giving you any new medicine, how often did hospital staff describe possible side effects in a way you could understand?	• Information, communication and education
Discharge information	During this hospital stay, did doctors, nurses or other hospital staff talk with you about whether you would have the help you needed when you left the hospital?	• Coordination and integration of care • Information, communication and education
	During this hospital stay, did doctors, nurses or other hospital staff talk with you about whether you would have the help you needed when you left the hospital?	• Coordination and integration of care • Information, communication and education
Hospital rating	Using any number from 0 to 10, where 0 is the worst hospital possible, and 10 is the best possible hospital, what number would you use to rate this hospital during your stay?	• All dimensions
Willingness to recommend hospital	Would you recommend this hospital to your family and friends?	• All dimensions
Care transition	During this hospital stay, staff took my preferences and those of my family or caregiver into account in deciding what my health care needs would be when I left.	• Involvement of family and friends • Coordination and integration of care

		• Respect for patients' values, preferences and expressed needs
	When I left the hospital, I had a good understanding of the things I was responsible for in managing my health.	• Coordination and integration of care • Information, communication and education
	When I left the hospital, I clearly understood the purpose for taking each of my medications.	• Coordination and integration of care • Information, communication and education

Table 2.1 – Picker Dimensions Mapped to HCAHPS questions

Although there is a lack of evidence in the literature suggesting the Picker Dimensions and HCAHPS are related, it is possible to map the HCAHPS questions to the Picker dimensions; however, as in the table above, each question can be mapped to more than one dimension. While the Picker dimensions help focus patient experience assessments as they relate to patient-centred care, the HCAHPS is a survey that uses a patient's perception of their hospital experience to assess satisfaction (Centers for Medicare & Medicaid Services, 2020). The HCAHPS intends to provide consumers with a method to rank care and provide health care administrators and researchers with areas of focus to improve healthcare services (Centers for Medicare & Medicaid Services, 2019). Consequently, the main focus of the HCAHPS is not to ensure that care is patient-centred instead, rather, it leverages patient experience to rank health systems.

Patient Experience Measurement in Canada

Canada has adopted similar assessment methods as the United States to improve healthcare delivery and outcomes (Canadian Institute for Health Information [CIHI], 2017). According to the Canadian Institute for Healthcare Improvement [CIHI] (2017), before 2016, patient experience was being measured inconsistently across Canada. There was a push to standardize patient experience measurement to compare Canadian healthcare jurisdictions (Canadian Institute for Health Information [CIHI], 2017). This push originated from CIHI's

Performance Measurement Framework for the Canadian Healthcare System, as one of its strategic priorities was measuring patient experience (Canadian Institute for Health Information [CIHI], 2013). The responsibility for healthcare delivery is provincial and territorial. Still, the universality, portability and accessibility criteria of the Canada Health Act generate expectations that health care provided across the country will be similar and provide similar results (Health Canada, 2015; Lanoix, 2017). Without standard measurement, it is difficult to determine that the health care provided produces equal outcomes across the country.

Canadian Patient Experience Survey – Inpatient Care

As a result of interprovincial/territorial work in 2017, CIHI released the Canadian Patient Experience Survey – Inpatient Care (CPES-IC) (Canadian Institute for Health Information [CIHI], 2017). It is a survey similar to the HCAHPS and uses the first twenty-two questions from the HCAHPS but adds nineteen additional questions to measure patient experience unique to the Canadian health care system (Canadian Institute for Health Information [CIHI], 2017). Table 2.2 provides a list of domains assessed by the HCAHPS and domains evaluated by the CPES-IC (Hadibhai, Lacroix, & Leeb, 2018). It is important to note that the HCAHPS domains have been updated since the release of the CPES-IC; see the previous section in this Chapter for the current HCAHPS domains. For example, pain control in the most recent HCAHPS has been replaced by care transition in the October 2019 version of the HCAHPS. The CPES-IC still has the original HCAHPS questions that assess pain control. For a current copy of the CPES-IC at the time of this work, please see Appendix B.

HCAHPS Domains (March 2018)	Additional CPES-IC Domains (January 2019)

• Communication with nurses
• Communication with doctors
• Physical environment
• Responsiveness of staff
• Pain control
	• Admission to hospital
	  ○ Direct admit
	  ○ Admit through emergency department
	• Internal coordination of care

• Communication about medications
• Discharge information
• Global hospital experience
  ○ Will recommend hospital
  ○ Hospital rating
	• Person-centred care
	  ○ Communication
	  ○ Timeliness of testing
	  ○ Involvement in decision-making
	  ○ Emotional support
	• Discharge and transition
	• Patient Safety
	• Outcome
	• Demographic
	• Global hospital experience
	  ○ Helped by hospital stay
	  ○ Overall hospital experience

Figure 2.1 – HCAHPS (March 2018) vs. CPES-IC Domains (January 2019)

The main focus of the CPES-IC is to provide hospital administrators in Canada with patient experience data for quality improvement (Canadian Institute for Health Information [CIHI], n.d.). Unlike the HCAHPS, the CPES-IC is not meant for consumers and instead is intended for hospitals to obtain improvement data. Specifically, it provides policy makers with a tool to compare and benchmark hospitals (Canadian Institute for Health Information [CIHI], n.d.). When examining the domains in Table 2.2, it should be noted that the CPES-IC does include patient experiences of patient-centred care, in contrast to the HCAHPS, which does not directly measure this (Hadibhai et al., 2018). While the CPES-IC has always measured transition and coordination of care, previous versions of the HCAHPS did not. However, the March 2020 version of the HCAHPS transition and coordination of care has now been included (Centers for Medicare & Medicaid Services, 2020).

The CPES-IC survey uses single or multiple questions to assess twenty-three different measures (Canadian Institute for Health Information [CIHI], 2019). These measures are more specific than the domains but maintain overlap with the survey questions. Table 2.3 provides the CPES-IC questions, which I mapped to CIHI's measures and domains. I mapped the measures and questions to the domains to demonstrate that measures and questions can provide information on more than one domain; however, there is little to no published literature combining the domains, measures, and questions (Hadibhai et al., 2018).

CPES-IC Question	CIHI Identified Measure	CIHI Identified Domain
• Was your admission into the hospital organized?	Admission into the Hospital (Direct Admission)	Admission to Hospital – Direct Admission
• During this hospital stay, how often were your room and bathroom kept clean?	Cleanliness	Physical Environment
• During this hospital stay, how often did doctors treat you with courtesy and respect? • During this hospital stay, how often did doctors listen carefully to you? • During this hospital stay, how often did doctors explain things in a way you could understand?	Communication with Doctors	Communication with Doctors Person Centred Care – Communication
• During this hospital stay, how often did nurses treat you with courtesy and respect? • During this hospital stay, how often did nurses listen carefully to you? • During this hospital stay, how often did nurses explain things in a way you could understand?	Communication with Nurses	Communication with Nurses Person Centred Care - Communication
• How often were tests and procedures done when you were told they would be done?	Coordination of Tests and Procedures	Internal Coordination of Care
• During this hospital stay, did doctors, nurses or other hospital staff talk with you about whether you would have the help you needed when you left the hospital? • During this hospital stay, did you get information in writing about what symptoms or health problems to look out for after you left the hospital?	Discharge Planning	Discharge Information Discharge and Transition
• Before you left the hospital, did you have a clear understanding about all of your prescribed medications, including those you were taking before your hospital stay? • Did you receive enough information from hospital staff about what to do if you were worried about your condition or treatment after you left the hospital? • When you left the hospital, did you have a better understanding of your condition than when you entered?	Discharge Management	Discharge and Transition Internal Coordination of Care

• Did you get the support you needed to help you with any anxieties, fears or worries you had during this hospital stay?	Emotional Support	Person Centred Care – Emotional Support
• Before coming to the hospital did you have enough information about what was going to happen during the admission process?	Enough Information Given About Admission Process, Prior to Arrival (Direct Admission)	Admission to Hospital – Direct Admission
• Before giving you any new medicine, how often did hospital staff tell you what the medicine was for? • Before giving you any new medicine, how often did hospital staff describe possible side effects in a way you could understand?	Explanation about Medications	Communication about medications Person Centred Care - Communication
• Using any number from 0 to 10, where 0 is the worst hospital possible and 10 is the best hospital possible, what number would you use to rate this hospital during your stay?	Hospital Rating (Worst to Best)	Global Hospital Experience – Hospital Rating
• Overall, do you feel you were helped by your hospital stay?	Hospital Stay Helpful	Global Hospital Experience – Hospital Stay Helpful
• When you were in the emergency department, did you get enough information about your condition and treatment? • Were you given enough information about what was going to happen during your admission to the hospital?	Information Shared with Patients in the Emergency Department (Admission through ED)	Person Centred Care – Communication Communication with nurses Communication with doctors
• Would you recommend this hospital to your friends and family?	Intent to Recommend Hospital to Family and Friends	Global Hospital Experience – will recommend hospital
• Do you feel that there was good communication about your care between doctors, nurses and other hospital staff? • How often did doctors, nurses and other hospital staff seem informed and up-to-date about your hospital care?	Internal Coordination of Care	Internal Coordination of Care
• Were you involved as much as you wanted to be in decisions about your care and treatment? • Were your family or friends involved as much as you wanted in decisions about your care and treatment?	Involvement in Decision Making	Person Centred Care – Involvement in Decision Making
• Overall... I had a very poor experience I had a very good experience (0 to 10 rating)	Overall Hospital Experience (Very poor to Very good)	Global Hospital Experience – Overall hospital experience

• During this hospital stay, how often was your pain well controlled? • During this hospital stay, how often did the hospital staff do everything they could to help you with your pain?	Pain Controlled	Pain Control
• During this hospital stay, how often was the area around your room quiet at night?	Quietness	Physical Environment
• During this hospital stay, did you get all the information you needed about your condition and treatment?	Received Information About Condition and Treatment	Person Centred Care – Communication
• During this hospital stay, after you pressed the call button, how often did you get help as soon as you wanted it? • How often did you get help in getting to the bathroom or in using a bedpan as soon as you wanted?	Staff Responsiveness	Responsiveness of Staff
• Was your transfer from the emergency department into a hospital bed organized?	Transfer from ED to Hospital Bed Organized (Admission through ED)	Admission to Hospital – admission through ED
• After you knew that you needed to be admitted to a hospital bed, did you have to wait too long before getting there?	Waiting Too Long in the ED for a Hospital Bed (Admission through ED)	Admission to Hospital – admission through ED

Table 2.2 – CPES-IC Measures to Topic Comparison

The CPES-IC questions are directly related to each measure. The CPES-IC domains may apply to more than one question. The focus of this work will use the CPES-IC measures instead of its domains as the domains are more narrowly focused in each question. More information about the methodology of this work is available in Chapter 4.

As the CPES-IC is still a newer survey and Canada has not previously had a national patient experience measurement survey, these measures and domains may change (Hadibhai et al., 2018). Although the CPES-IC has been endorsed by Accreditation Canada as a survey to meet accreditation requirements, hospitals are not required to administer it at this time (Canadian Institute for Health Information [CIHI], n.d.). However, should these requirements change in the future, the CPES-IC does have the potential to measure hospitals' performance. Some of the limiting factors preventing this are whether or not case-mix and patient variables affect the survey results, which has occurred with HCAHPS results (Hadibhai et al., 2018). However, unlike its American counterpart, the Canadian survey does hold potential to improve patient-centred care and ensure care delivered is similar across the nation.

Patient-centred Care, Patient Experience, Patient Satisfaction and the Relationship with Performance Measurement

As mentioned earlier in this Chapter, patient experience can measure patient-centred care. However, the relationships between patient-centred care, patient experience and patient satisfaction are important to understand when measuring performance. A recent framework (Figure 2.2) by Larson et al. (2019) has demonstrated the relationship between patient-centred care, patient experience and patient satisfaction.

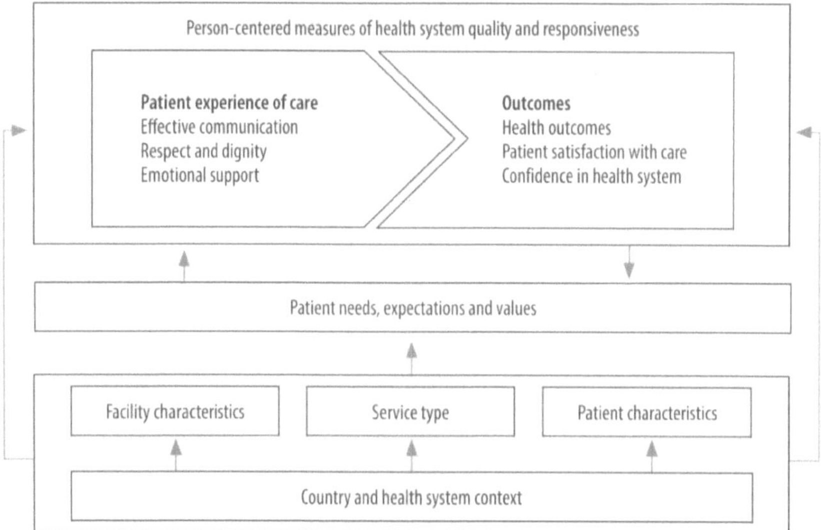

Figure 2.2 – Larson et al. (2019) Framework for person-centred measures of health system quality
and responsiveness. Taken from This is an open access ~~article distributed under the terms of the Creative Commons~~ Attribution IGO License (which permits unrestricted use, distribution, and reproduction in any medium, provided the original work is properly cited. In any reproduction of this article there should not be any suggestion that WHO or this article endorse any specific organization or products. The use of the WHO logo is not permitted. This notice should be preserved along with the article's original URL

The authors describe patient experience as a process measure for patient-centred care, where the patient's experience is used to ensure that activities designed to improve care are taking place. Using patient experience this way helps demonstrate health system accountability or the quality of care delivered. However, Larson et al. (2019) also suggest that the patient experience can also capture patient satisfaction. Satisfaction is an expression that reflects an outcome of the service received captured through the patient experience (Larson et al., 2019). Measurement of patient-centred care requires capturing both process and outcome of an intervention. Together these help determine how patient-centred an intervention may be. For example, suppose a nurse administers an ad hoc medication at a patient's request knowing it will only make the patient happy. Although the patient may be satisfied with this intervention, the care was not patient-centred as the medication may not have been warranted. Similarly, if a nurse coerced administering an ad hoc medication to ensure best practice but did not consider the patient's wishes, this also indicates a lack of patient-centredness. While the nurse may have adhered to best practice, the patient may not have been satisfied with the interaction as they were not provided a choice. Suppose the nurse offers the same medication but provides a rationale for its administration. In this scenario, regardless of whether the patient accepts or does not want the drug, the patient receives patient-centred care. This is indicated as the medication is best practice, and the outcome is congruent with the patient's wishes. In the examples above, patient experience is used as a proxy to measure patient-centred care. However, it is vital to ensure that any measure is tested and validated, primarily if used as a performance measure.

Performance Measurement

In healthcare jurisdictions worldwide, small experiments have begun to determine if the measurement of patient experience and associated improvements with a patient's health outcomes should be tied to financial incentives (Elliott et al., 2016; Stanowski, Simpson, & White, 2015). In the United States, where healthcare funding is increasingly tied to health outcomes, there is a push to ensure that experiences that improve outcomes are delivered (McWilliams, Landon, Chernew, & Zaslavsky, 2014). As healthcare costs have increased, the value received from health care services has not increased in kind. Much of healthcare is currently paid through volume-based incentives where increased patient throughput and services delivered equates with financial remuneration. While this does improve the number of patients seen, it has not improved health outcomes. To meet the triple aim, values and outcomes-based financial incentives have been proposed to reduce cost and improve outcomes. No longer is it sufficient to only treat patients. Health systems are becoming accountable for the costs of treatments and the outcomes of those treatments. Unfortunately, similar to volume-based incentives where the objective is to improve throughput, outcomes-based incentives can suffer similar pitfalls where populations are excluded, or metrics are manipulated to improve remuneration or prevent penalties.

Many measures that are used to reward or penalize specific behaviours often succumb to Campbell's law, in which "the more any quantitative social indicator is used for social decision-making, the more subject it will be to corruption pressures and the more apt it will be to distort and corrupt the social processes it is intended to monitor" (Campbell, 1979 p. 67). Baker & Qaseem (2011) and Mannion & Braithwaite (2012) have noticed that using metrics to reward or penalize performance tends to introduce unintended consequences such as: measurement fixation, which is the tendency to ensure targets are met at the expense of actual benefit to the patient or health care system; or quantification privileging, which is the reduction of complex phenomena to numbers as opposed to using mixed methods to quantify the phenomena (Mannion

& Braithwaite, 2012). Although there have been proposed strategies to mitigate these, biases will always exist.

There has been evidence of this happening within Canada already. In the early 2010s, the British Columbia (BC) Ministry of Health tried to reduce emergency departments' access times. Although not entirely conclusive, Wang, Ding, Park, & Hunte (2019) discovered some evidence that pay-for-performance measures designed to improve access to health care services may have inadvertently increased readmission rates. In the late 2000s, CIHI introduced the Hospital Standardized Mortality Ratio (HSMR), which allowed for comparison of in-hospital death rates (Canadian Institute for Health Information [CIHI], 2007). On the year of the release of this score, a hospital in BC was determined to have one of the country's highest HSMR scores (Anderson, 2007). There was a public inquiry into the cause, and it was determined that inaccurate coding led to data submissions that may have accounted for a higher than average HSMR. Rather than continue to investigate other potential causes, the proposed solution was to fix the coding errors that ended up removing patients who could have inflated the HSMR scores. Chong, Nguyen, & Wilcox (2012) have noted that removing specific patient population data from the HSMR metrics has caused an overall improvement in the HSMR score over time. This outcome may have been unintentional; however, it is an example of the unintended consequence of health care jurisdictions trying to improve their score by focusing on improving a single metric.

Preventing Unintended Consequences

Sidorkin (2016) stated that changing an organization's culture to ensure that it is not opposed to measurement is one way to ensure that unintended consequences occur less often. Braithwaite (2018) notes that culture shifts do not happen quickly, nor are they easily predictable within a health care setting. Data triangulation and determining alternate methods to reach similar endpoints have been discussed by Baker & Qaseem (2011) as methods that can reduce the problems introduced by using metrics for performance. Carter, Bryant-Lukosius, Dicenso, Blythe, & Neville (2014) have indicated that triangulation can be used to determine data validity across multiple sources. However, Carter et al. (2014) also noted that this method is limited by the ability to obtain data from numerous sources. The use of crowd-sourced[2] information on social media platforms has been suggested as one potential source for data triangulation (Dai, Mausam, & Weld, 2010).

Social media as an adjunct to traditional quality surveys has been proposed by Ranard et al. (2016) to supplement conventional quality surveys. The authors suggest that similar information is contained in social media reviews that can also be found on the HCAHPS survey. Using natural language processing techniques, the authors provided evidence that social media reviews could be used as an alternate source of information. It is feasible that social media mining can supplement survey data to ensure that policy and decision-makers have another data source to ensure surveys are not manipulated. However, processes and infrastructure would need to be developed to leverage social media as a data source for quality. While these techniques have been used less often in health care, other industries have leveraged social media's power to improve and promote their services.

Social Media Mining

Salehan & Kim (2016) and Zhang, Cheng, Liao, & Choudhary (2011) have noted that obtaining information from social media websites can provide valuable information to improve

---

[2] Crowd-sourced refers to obtaining information, work or opinions from data submitted to the internet, social media or other applications. See Dai, Mausam & Weld (2010) for additional information

commercial products and services. In recent years, studies on this phenomenon in health care have increased. Abualigah, Alfar, Shehab, & Hussein (2020); Marsh, Peacock, Sheard, Hughes, & Lawton (2019), and Soto et al. (2018) have all suggested how data can be used to capture the patient experience and be used for determining areas to improve healthcare quality. They state the most significant challenge with utilizing social media data is that most data are not readily consumable.

The reviews may apply to various contexts and time points within a health care encounter, making it more challenging to determine how or when to use the findings. One of the examples brought up by Lyles & Sarkar (2013) was that data could apply to an entire visit, including how difficult it was to find parking or food quality in the cafeteria. Lyles & Sarkar (2013) determined that some data may not be applicable in the quality improvement of a service. Other challenges also exist, such as deliberate attempts at gaming[3], sample and selection bias, using this type of data (Greaves, Ramirez-Cano, Millett, Darzi, & Donaldson, 2013). Similarly, context can be lost when categorizing or organizing the data due to aggregation by natural language processing (Lyles & Sarkar, 2013).

Researchers have noted that it is crucial to understand how data is analyzed to use data appropriately (Lyles & Sarkar, 2013; Marsh et al., 2019; Soto et al., 2018). Social media information should not be used as the sole source of information due to the challenges mentioned previously, but should be combined with other types of evaluative methods to ensure accuracy. Although it is not recommended to use social media data as a primary source of information, it can help narrow down or pinpoint other topics of interest that could be used for further study.

[3] A deliberate attempt to follow the rules but focus on activities that improve a metric or score while reducing focus on activities that do not count toward a score. See Morreim (1991) for additional examples and definition of gaming.

Wang, Xu, Fujita, & Liu (2016) noted difficulties using big data[4] to make decisions. Ensuring accuracy requires personnel who understand and interpret the data correctly and proper infrastructure to understand the data. Without these critical aspects to operate a big data program, the data as well as invested time and money may be unhelpful or useless (Wang et al., 2016).

Social Media and Improvement in Other Industries

Social media review data has not been utilized as heavily in healthcare as in other industries. It has been touted by Hajli (2014), Kärkkäinen, Jussila, & Väisänen (2010), and Rathore, Ilavarasan, & Dwivedi (2016) as a method to capture feedback in an efficient and timely manner. For example, when determining how best to improve a product or service, Rathore et al. (2016) have demonstrated that social media can improve subsequent versions of the product. This includes both physical items as well as versions of software. Social media reviews have also become a way to determine if a service is worth utilizing in the service industry. Kim, Li, & Brymer (2016) have shown that consumers' social media use has driven these businesses to improve their quality to ensure the total number of reviews and each reviewer's score is high. Erkan & Evans (2016) have also demonstrated that a business' social media review score can impact a consumer's intention to purchase or utilize a service. Although not directly related to health care quality, it is hypothesized that consumer behaviours could also extend to healthcare (Grabner-Kräuter & Waiguny, 2015). Unfortunately, further research in this area is still required to determine how much and what components of an online review influence a patient's intention to utilize a health care service (Schulz & Rothenfluh, 2020). Schulz &

[4] Big data refers to the size, complexity and speed data is available. For additional information and definitions see Wang, Xu, Fujita & Liu (2016).

Rothenfluh (2020) determined that reading social media reviews of health care providers affected choice in seeing a provider and the patient's attitude toward and perception of that provider's skill. While the evidence is emerging that intention to use services is affected by social media reviews, many health care systems are not adapted and need to develop processes to incorporate these sources of data within their quality improvement repertoire (Grabner-Kräuter & Waiguny, 2015). Unfortunately, health care in Canada has not widely adopted social media data to improve care quality at a system level (De Angelis et al., 2018).

Nurses and Information Technology

Nurses comprise the largest workforce in health care, particularly within the acute care setting, where nursing care directly affects patients' experience and outcomes. Nurses are in the best position to ensure that quality care is provided. However, Dempsey, Reilly, & Buhlman (2014) have noted that nurses, particularly those at the point of care, are constrained in many ways from being engaged in improving the quality of their care. The highest engagement and commitment to improving care peaks at around six months after graduation and does not improve unless a nurse transitions to an administrative role. While personal factors may affect a nurse's ability to be engaged, system-wide challenges often prevent nurses from meaningful engagement (Goldman et al., 2018). Van Bogaert, Kowalski, Weeks, Van Heusden, & Clarke (2013) have noticed that point of care nurses do not receive opportunities to be part of decision-making processes, nor are they exposed to the data which may help them improve their care. For example, Goldman et al. (2018) have found that issues with interprofessional practice and inclusion during patient rounds have been seen as one such area. Point of care nurses often are not included in discharge planning, and this results in a suboptimal patient experience as nurses are sometimes surprised by the plan of care. Despite knowing about the challenge, the inclusion of point of care nurses in quality improvement is difficult due to financial and time constraints. particularly in Canada, where most healthcare dollars are spent on staffing with little room for extras. Information technology, has the promise to make it easier for staff to be both engaged and reduce some of the system inequities in nurses work.

Combining natural language processing and readily available free-text user reviews holds promise to engage direct care nurses and other health care providers in the use of data to improve care (Ranard et al., 2016). The use of aggregated social media data can provide data on the care nurses, and other interprofessional team members provide a patient on a particular unit or service (Ranard et al., 2016). Unfortunately, most health care jurisdictions do not currently have the resources to take advantage of this readily available data (Ranard et al., 2016). However, the use of natural language processing algorithms has turned a once labour and time-intensive task of collating, analyzing and aggregating data into a process that can be cost-efficient, repeatable and reliable depending on what type of information the algorithm is programmed to aggregate. Discussion of natural language processing and its benefits is discussed briefly in Chapter 3. In general, natural language processing of free-text reviews can address the barrier of access to data.

Gaps in the Literature

The literature reviewed suggests that social media reviews can be used as an adjunct to traditional survey methods. However, evidence for this is lacking in the Canadian context. It has been demonstrated that measuring a patient's experience can be a proxy measure for determining how patient-centred care is, as long as the measures are designed to provide data on what it is being intended to measure. Survey tools measuring the quality of care alone may prove harmful if used for decision-making or evaluative purposes without triangulating other sources of information. This has been particularly highlighted when incentives or penalties are associated with results. Therefore, using alternate methods to capture data about the same phenomenon may help determine if what is being measured is actually measured.

Data capture using surveys and focus groups can be costly due to the number of persons who can participate and the financial costs to capture and analyze this data. Already a staple in other service industries, the use of readily available social media data has the ability to supplement traditional surveys. Although this remains a gap in the Canadian context, using social media data sources may validate and supplement traditional survey methods. While traditional survey methods allow longitudinal tracking of changes over time, these may not capture items patients themselves feel are important. This is particularly important in patient-centred care, as one dimension of patient-centred care is that patients' values, wishes, and expressed needs are respected. Repeated surveys can quickly adapt to assessing values, wishes and needs that change. Given health care that is patient-centred and includes the values and preferences of patients has been shown to improve patient outcomes, it is important to ensure that patients participate and provide feedback as well as discuss areas of their care that they feel are important. Therefore, the research questions guiding this research may help address the gaps identified in this literature review:

1) Do Google free-text user reviews of hospitals in British Columbia contain information captured in domains of the Canadian Patient Experience Survey – Inpatient Care?
2) Do these same free-text user reviews also contain information not captured in the domains of the Canadian Patient Experience Survey – Inpatient Care?

Chapter 3 – Latent Dirichlet Allocation

Introduction

This Chapter will provide a brief overview of Latent Dirichlet Allocation (LDA). The intent is to provide the reader with a brief history, describe how it operates, and provide rationale and limitations for its use.

What is Latent Dirichlet Allocation (LDA)?

LDA is a generative probabilistic model that can derive topics from large sets of discrete data (Blei, Ng, & Jordan, 2003). In the domain of machine learning, LDA has been used to identify and categorize patterns within discrete data that would be difficult to complete by a human alone (Jacobi, Van Atteveldt, & Welbers, 2016). The use of LDA provides the ability to quickly identify themes or topics from a large set of data after the initial seeding of the model with parameters. The following example will be used throughout this Chapter to clarify some of the abstract concepts with LDA.

LDA Case Example – Finding Five Books of Interest

Imagine one has to select five books to read from a one thousand book collection. Unfortunately, these books have not been previously catalogued, nor are there dust jackets that summarize or provide a glimpse inside each book. Although one could easily select five books randomly, for this example, imagine one would like to read five books of interest. Without an easy way to determine the topics within each book, selection could be based on titles of interest. However, a title is not always indicative of the content contained within a book and selecting books using this method may likely provide reading that is not of interest. Another approach may be to choose books at random or via some defined pattern and browse through them. While a possible strategy, without previous categorizations or other information this may be time-consuming or increase the possibility that one would miss many other books of interest.

How does LDA work?

Using LDA may provide an alternate method of book selection. LDA uses the power of statistics, computer programming and computer processing that work together to give a topic list across all books and identify topics contained within individual books (Maier et al., 2018).

Using the book example above, LDA works by having a computer calculate the statistical probabilities that words (or other discrete data) appear together (Maier et al., 2018). Data must be cleaned and readied before LDA processing (Nikolenko, Koltcov, & Koltsova, 2017). Cleaning data can be completed via other computer programs that help prepare data for LDA.

1) The content of each book must be loaded into a computer program
2) All punctuation must be removed
3) All capital letters become lower case
4) All stop words are removed (pronouns, prepositions, terms that should not be part of the analysis)
5) Remaining words are stemmed – returned to root word (e.g. politics, politician, political = politi)

These steps allow the computer to easily count words and perform statistical analysis on the word groupings (Schofield, Magnusson, Thompson, & Mimno, 2017).

Unfortunately, LDA cannot suggest how many word groupings exist within the data set as this must be determined by the user running the analysis (Hecking & Leydesdorff, 2019). LDA analysis can also not provide the topic names; instead, it gives the user common word groupings. In this way, each analysis using LDA can be unique if different parameters are applied or data is cleaned differently (Hecking & Leydesdorff, 2019). However, once the analysis is complete, it provides statistical analysis for each book's topics and across all books (Blei et al., 2003). In this way, it can help establish which books contain similar topics and which books are unrelated.

Returning to the example, if the topic of 'outer space' is identified, LDA can help group which books most likely have 'outer space' as a topic. If one was interested in outer space, the book search could be narrowed to the books with the highest probabilities of containing the topic of outer space. Perhaps the search for outer space books has refined the one thousand books to two hundred related to outer space. While significantly reducing the number of books to browse, this would take a long time to narrow to a specific topic of interest. Suppose one wanted to find books related to the planet Jupiter specifically. In this case, it is possible to run another LDA analysis of the identified books to determine which books have the planet Jupiter as a topic, narrowing the focus area. It would be possible to search for Jupiter in the one thousand book collection, however without limiting the scope first; the results may be more challenging to interpret as Jupiter could be used in contents outside of 'outer space'. For example, Jupiter could refer to the Roman god, an island near Florida or a type of grape. One could also attempt a general word search on the first set of topics identified by LDA; however, searching this way would search on outer space topics, which may not be directly related to the planet Jupiter. While you could use a word search on the planet Jupiter of the remaining two hundred books, there is still a possibility of obtaining non-specific results. Instead of finding non-fiction literature on the planet Jupiter, it is entirely possible to find a fiction book about the planet Jupiter. Completing a secondary analysis on the two hundred books would provide a more specific topic listing contained within each book and hopefully yield reference books with the planet Jupiter as a topic.

In a literature search, sensitivity and specificity are crucial concepts to consider. As these concepts are inversely related, as the specificity of a search increases, the sensitivity decreases. It is necessary to find a balance between both measures to ensure an optimal literature search. In the examples from above, using LDA helps find a list of relevant books faster than a traditional word search might. Given that LDA will provide a grouping of words relevant to each book, it may prove to be quicker in finding relevant books than searching for single terms and manually filtering through each. While searching for individual words may increase sensitivity, there will also be many results unrelated to the topic of interest. Searching for both outer space, the planet Jupiter, and other characteristics of the planet Jupiter may improve a search's specificity. However, this may dramatically decrease the number of books overall, potentially eliminating other books relevant to the topic of interest. Using LDA may help obtain that balance between specificity and sensitivity to help find topics faster than traditional search methods.

LDA: A Little More Detail

Although the example above with books might help understand the process at a high level, the following example will describe how LDA identifies topics. Suppose one had five outer space-related sentences. Table 3.1 below illustrates how completing the LDA process may render the sentences with a comparison between the original and my interpretation of what LDA may do to the sentences. Following the steps to complete LDA analysis removing common language words is fundamental as these can change the distribution of words. Punctuation and capitalization will also be removed, leaving the following words in each sentence. The words will not be stemmed to maintain context for the reader.

	Original Sentence	LDA Interpreted Sentence
Sentence 1	Jupiter has a giant red spot.	jupiter giant red spot
Sentence 2	Jupiter is a large gas giant.	jupiter large gas giant
Sentence 3	Earth's surface is rocky but is mainly covered in water.	earth surface rocky mainly covered water
Sentence 4	Earth has rocky mountains.	earth rocky mountain
Sentence 5	The gas giant Jupiter is so large, you can see it from Earth's surface without being on a rocky mountain.	gas giant jupiter large earth surface rocky mountain

Table 3.1 – Example sentences and example sentences converted for LDA

I will attempt to use a graphical representation to illustrate what might happen when LDA is completed on the converted sentences in table 3.1. Table 3.2 below demonstrates each sentence's topic relatedness that might be seen when running LDA analysis, assuming a distribution of words about two pre-selected topics. For this example, I have pre-selected the two topics: Earth and Jupiter. LDA will not identify the topics, only groupings of words. Please see the Limitations section later in this Chapter for additional information on this.

	Sentence 1	Sentence 2	Sentence 3	Sentence 4	Sentence 5
Total # of Words	4	4	6	3	8
Words	jupiter giant red spot	jupiter large gas giant	earth surface rocky mainly covered water	earth rocky mountain	gas giant jupiter large earth surface rocky mountain
Probability of each topic	100% Jupiter	100% Jupiter	100% Earth	100% Earth	50% Jupiter 50% Earth

Table 3.2 – Example probability of topics related to each sentence

To further understand the table above results, LDA operates off a probabilistic model that relates words to each other. Taking all five sentences nets the following matrixes of words below in figure 3.1

Sentence 1 v. Sentence 2

	jupiter	giant	red	spot
jupiter	x			
large				
gas				
giant		x		

Sentence 1 v. Sentence 5

	gas	giant	jupiter	large	earth	surface	rocky	mountain
jupiter			x					
giant		x						
red								
spot								

Sentence 2 v. Sentence 5

	gas	giant	jupiter	large	earth	surface	rocky	mountain
jupiter			x					
large				x				
gas	x							
giant		x						

Sentence 2 v. Sentence 4

	earth	rocky	mountain
jupiter			
large			
gas			
giant			

Sentence 1 v. Sentence 4

	earth	rocky	mountain
jupiter			
giant			
red			
spot			

Sentence 3 v. Sentence 4

	earth	surface	rocky	mainly	covered	water
earth	X					
rocky			x			
mountain						

Sentence 4 v. Sentence 5

	gas	giant	jupiter	large	earth	surface	rocky	mountain
earth					x			
rocky							x	
mountain								x

Sentence 3 v. Sentence 5

	gas	giant	jupiter	large	earth	surface	rocky	mountain
earth					x			
surface						x		
rocky							x	
mainly								
covered								
water								

Sentence 3 v. Sentence 1

	jupiter	giant	red	spot
earth				
surface				
rocky				
mainly				
covered				
water				

Sentence 3 v. Sentence 2

	jupiter	large	gas	giant
earth				
surface				
rocky				
mainly				
covered				
water				

Figure 3.1 – Example Simplified LDA Probability Matrix

The figure's purpose is to demonstrate how LDA will analyze the words contained in each sentence and show how sentences could be related to one another. An 'x' in a box indicates that the two compared sentences share a word between them. Examining the breakdown of figure 3.1, Sentences 1 and 2 share words, as do sentences 3 and 4, indicating that these sentences' pairings are related. Both sentences 1 and 2 also share words with sentence 5, likewise sentences 3 and 4 also share words with sentence 5, indicating both pairings are related to sentence 5. Note that sentences 2 & 4, 1 & 3, 2 & 3, and 1 & 4 have no similarities between them and are likely unrelated. Of note, sentence 5 shares six words with sentences 1 & 2 and 3 & 4, indicating they are of equal relation. Looking at only the words that matched across the five sentences, LDA would likely output the following word groupings:

Topic A: Jupiter, giant, gas, large

Topic B: Earth, rocky, mountain, surface

Examining the topic list generated, a LDA user could interpret these as Jupiter and Earth, although other topics are possible. The previous example is a simplification, and it does illustrate how LDA works. However, given that LDA analysis was meant to be completed on data sets many times larger than the example, showing this across an extensive collection could not be done briefly. Specifically, the example cannot discuss how the identification of topic number drives the analysis and determines the groupings of words that form topics.

LDA: Perplexity and Coherence Scoring and Topic Inference

The topic number is LDA analysis's cornerstone (Hecking & Leydesdorff, 2019). It provides the computer with the necessary parameters to determine groupings of words. However, computers cannot judge the analysis results and therefore cannot offer inferences into what groupings of words yield the best topics. Therefore, a human is still required to interpret the data and provide meaning to the groupings of words and label them as a topic. Using the previous example for topics, imagine if the number of topics selected for the analysis was six rather than two. The following topic list may be generated:

Topic A: Jupiter, large	Topic B: Gas	Topic C: Giant	Topic D: Earth	Topic E: surface	Topic F: rocky, mountains

Table 3.3 – Example of six topic LDA on the data set

As the number of topics selected increases, there is a change in context. The computer is now looking for more groupings and identifying statistical relationships between the higher numbers of topics. To combat this difficulty identifying the number of topics, users of LDA have developed two metrics that can aid judgement in topic number selection: coherence and perplexity scoring (Ghosh & Guha, 2013; Jacobi et al., 2016; Rosner, Hinneburg, Röder, Nettling, & Both, 2014). However, regardless of the scores, it's important to note that human judgement must still be exercised to determine topic number feasibility.

Coherence scoring and perplexity scoring help provide metrics that determine how interpretable a grouping of words might be. Coherence scores determine how interpretable the word groupings might be; whereas, perplexity scoring helps determine how random the word groupings might be (Rosner et al., 2014). Therefore, low perplexity and high coherence are preferable given that high coherence indicates the word groupings are understandable, and low perplexity means the word groupings are less random. Returning to the previous example with the topics nets the table below:

# of Topics	2	6	8
Topic A	Jupiter, gas, giant, large	Jupiter, large	Jupiter
Topic B	Earth, rocky, mountain, surface	Gas	Large
Topic C		Giant	Gas
Topic D		Earth	Giant
Topic E		Surface	Earth
Topic F		Rocky, mountain	surface

Topic G			Rocky
Topic H			mountain

Table 3.4 – Example of perplexity and coherence on ascending topic numbers

It can be seen that as the topic number increases, the context of the word groupings is lost. However, the higher the topic number, the less judgement required to determine the topic. In this example, the two topics may provide a higher coherence score meaning they are easier to understand; however, perplexity compared with topics six and eight may be higher or more random. Conversely, topics six and eight may have lower perplexity scores, but due to lack of groupings, the coherence is low and not as easy to understand. As each topic's words become more specific with the higher topic number categories, it is less likely the word groupings are random. Although a user could infer topic names from any of the topic number examples above, having a priori knowledge of the subject aids in interpretation of the groupings (Chen, Mukherjee, Liu, Hsu, & Castellanos, 2013).

Limitations of LDA

As mentioned previously in this Chapter, LDA analysis relies on identifying a fixed number of topics. Although a dataset may hold many topics, setting the topic number allows the algorithm to determine which words most likely correlate across all documents related to the topic number selected (Blei et al., 2003). Returning to the book example and the search for the planet Jupiter, if only one book discussed the planet Jupiter, selecting a small topic number such as ten may not result in any topics related to Jupiter as other topics may appear. This could also hold if no books in the set contained information on the planet Jupiter. In practice, one generally will only investigate a dataset that may provide positive results unless the investigation is entirely exploratory. According to Roitblat (2020), LDA is characterized as identifying topics present in 80% of a dataset where the remaining 20% of documents he claims can be misclassified. Roitblat (2020) found no topics were missed across the entire dataset, even in the misclassified data. A caveat to this work is that his dataset already had a fixed number of pre-identified topics, which means.that he was not attempting to find the correct topic number or trying to discover new topics. Instead, his LDA analysis focused on determining if any pre-identified topics were missed. This work does bring additional credence to the importance of a priori knowledge of a subject and the importance of human-computer interaction.

Importance of Human Interaction

Although LDA is a powerful tool that can only be completed via computer, the computer itself is insufficient to complete the analysis. Likewise, a human cannot comprehend the amount of data a computer can parse given the same amount of time. The use of LDA highlights the importance of both the computer and human, as the computer facilitates the processing of information promptly. Although any human may be able to provide meaning to the computer's outputs for LDA, the process of completing LDA and refining the analysis is made easier if the person conducting the analysis has pre-existing knowledge of the subject (Chen et al., 2013). While anyone could run an LDA analysis on any subject of interest, the analysis may be more straightforward if someone knows the subject area. For example, taking the topic of this book, someone without knowledge of quality measures in Canadian health care may be unable to interpret or recreate the data obtained in this book as differences in ideas, opinions and thoughts between the readers of this book and myself may exist.

Chapter 4 – Methods

Introduction

The methods discussed in this Chapter were used to answer the following research questions:

1) Do Google free-text user reviews of hospitals in British Columbia contain information captured in domains of the Canadian Patient Experience Survey – Inpatient Care?
2) Do these same free-text user reviews also contain information not captured in the domains of the Canadian Patient Experience Survey – Inpatient Care?

It is important to note that although the methods between this book and the study by Ranard et al. (2016) may be similar, the health systems of the two countries and the survey tools differ, which may affect the research outcomes. Details on the Ranard et al. (2016) study are provided below. Comparison of the Canadian Patient Experience Survey – Inpatient Care (CPES-IC) and the Hospital Consumer Assessment of Healthcare Providers and Systems (HCAHPS) are in Chapter 2. As the use of natural language processing methods to generate topics from free-text social media reviews has not been widely adopted in Canadian healthcare, this study's focus is exploratory.

Background

Ranard et al. (2016) compared the Hospital Consumer Assessment of Healthcare Providers and Systems (HCAHPS) survey to online Yelp reviews of hospitals. Yelp is an American company that hosts and markets a website that publishes crowd-sourced reviews for businesses (Yelp.com, 2021b). Businesses can be listed on the website by users to write a review about that business (Yelp.com, 2021a). Owners or operators can claim the business to use the Yelp website to interact with users (Yelp.com, 2021a). Ranard et. al's (2016) study comparison was completed by using natural language processing methods to obtain topics from word groupings and then comparing the identified topics to the domains from the HCAHPS. The word groupings were determined using latent dirichlet allocation (LDA), a type of natural language processing that groups words automatically, and the researchers manually labeling each grouping of words. When these labels were contrasted against domains from the HCAHPS, the researchers found that Yelp reviews contained information found in the HCAHPS as well as additional domains not found within the HCAHPS.

Design

Similar to the study above, a non-experimental comparative design was used to address the research questions. Twenty-three CIHI measures were utilized as topics to compare with emergent topics identified using Latent Dirichlet Allocation (LDA) of Google user reviews of 94 hospitals in BC. A list of the measures found in the CPES-IC is identified in Figure 4.1 below (Canadian Institute for Health Information [CIHI], 2019). For the LDA comparison, the measures were used as topics to compare against groupings of words found by LDA analysis.

<table>
<tr><th>All Admissions</th><th>Direct Admissions</th></tr>
<tr><td rowspan="3">• Cleanliness
• Communication with Doctors
• Communication with Nurses
• Coordination of Tests and Procedures
• Discharge Planning
• Discharge Management
• Emotional Support
• Explanation about Medications
• Hospital Rating (Worst to Best)
• Hospital Stay Helpful
• Intent to Recommend Hospital to Family or Friends
• Internal Coordination of Care
• Involvement in Decision-Making
• Overall Hospital Experience (Very Poor to Very Good)
• Pain Controlled
• Quietness
• Received Information about Treatment and Condition
• Staff Responsiveness</td><td>• Enough Information Given about Admission Process Prior to Arrival
• Admission to Hospital Organized</td></tr>
<tr><td>Admissions Through ED</td></tr>
<tr><td>• Information Shared with patients in the Emergency Department
• Waiting Too Long in the ED for a Hospital Bed
• Transfer from ED to Hospital Bed Organized</td></tr>
</table>

Figure 4.1 – Topics from CPES-IC as identified by CIHI (2019, March)

Ethics

Approval for this study was obtained from the University of Victoria Human Ethics Research Board on September 14, 2020 (protocol #19-0383). Data collection commenced after approval was obtained.

Confidentiality

The data being used for this research is readily available on the web, making it accessible to anyone interested in the data and connection to the internet. However, I did not collect user-identifying information, and the data was aggregated, making it difficult to identify a specific individual's user review. Any other possibly identifying information in the body of a review remained, but this was secured as discussed earlier in the section on data storage and has not been included as part of this work.

Consent

Consent was not required as Google's terms of service do not prohibit the use of user reviews for research (Google.com, 2020b). By publishing a user review, a user provides Google with the permission to share the content unless the posting user revokes the review or the review is flagged as inappropriate and removed by a Google moderator (Google.com, 2020a).

Use of Data

Other than using the research data as outlined in this Chapter to complete and publish this book on UVic Space, I do not anticipate any other uses of this data. However, this does not exclude the possibility in the future that portions of this book may be published in relevant journals or disseminated at professional conferences or seminars.

Conflict of Interest

During the period this research was conducted, I was employed by the agencies that own and operate the hospitals being researched. However, my employment was unrelated to quality improvement and patient experience at these hospitals. I have no other conflicts of interest to declare.

Data Collection

Hospital Selection Criteria

Reviews for acute care hospitals listed on the Hospital Address List on the Government of British Columbia's (BC) Finding Hospitals, Clinics and Doctors webpage were included (Province of BC, 2017). Extended care facilities, diagnostic and treatment-only centres, and hospitals in the miscellaneous section of the list were excluded from data collection as these were not considered acute care hospitals on the Province of BC's list. Although hospitals across Canada could have been included in this research, hospitals in BC were selected for proof of concept.

Google Reviews

Google reviews were selected because this type of research did not violate the terms of the user agreement and ensured enough user reviews were available to conduct the analysis (Google.com, 2020b). As mentioned in Chapter 3, although there are no standard criteria required to complete the LDA analysis, a higher number of documents generally improves the related words in identified domains (Crossley, Dascalu, & Mcnamara, 2017).

All user reviews posted to the Google review web address for each hospital were included on the date they were abstracted. There were no criteria that suggested excluding specific data would limit the analysis in this exploratory design.

A GNU public license python program was modified to facilitate downloading the hospital reviews in preparation for analysis (github.com, 2019 June 11). The program was modified from a script posted to github.com that previously downloaded a fixed number of reviews. The python program was altered to abstract all reviews, including:

1) The date of the review;
2) The body of the review; and
3) The web address of the review.

The script was fed the web address of each hospital's Google reviews web address. The web addresses had to be manually added to the script. Images, "likes," and scores were excluded from the data capture as they were not relevant to this research design. Although images posted to Google reviews may contain context pertinent to a user's review, they were excluded as the method of LDA being employed operates on text only. "Likes," while important in communicating to other readers that a review may be a favourite, did not provide information relevant to this design, so they were also excluded. The overall score indicates satisfaction with the hospital; however, overall scores were not compared, so these were excluded. As the LDA analysis relied on reading all reviews in a single file, each hospital's reviews were saved in a single comma-separated values (CSV) file. Each hospital was denoted by its web address.

Ninety-four Google review web addresses yielded 4,642 reviews for download. Table 4.2 provides basic statistics about the downloaded data set.

Total Reviews	Average Words	Median Words	Maximum Words	Minimum Words	Standard Deviation
4,644	65.03	39	1,446	1	84.4

Table 4.1 – Descriptive Statistics about downloaded reviews

Data Storage

The data were stored on my personal computer. The computer was password protected and required biometric authentication to access. The folder containing the data is only accessible to me. The folder is not accessible to any cloud-based applications. Five years after this work is accepted, I will securely remove the folder containing the data from the personal computer by using an application that overwrites the sectors of the hard drive where the research data is held multiple times. The five-year timeline has been selected to preserve the data if there is a request to access the original data set.

Data Preparation

The data were prepared using a modification of the standard LDA data preparation procedure outlined in Chapter 3 of this work because of additional non-alphanumeric characters within the data. Python command line was used to prepare the data. The data were prepared per the protocol below:

1) All letters were made lowercase
2) All punctuation was removed
3) Stop words were removed
4) Emoticons were removed
5) Emojis were removed
6) Any remaining non-alphanumeric characters were removed

7) Remaining text in reviews were lemmatized

An example of the code used to prepare the data is Appendix C. Lemmatization was selected instead of stemmatization due to the ability to map words to root words instead of removing the participle's tense. While word stemming and lemmatization are similar in that these linguistic techniques transform words into a format that is easier to process, there are several differences (Brahmi, Ech-Cherif, & Benyettou, 2012). Stemming a word removes suffixes but does not transform words, where lemmatization not only eliminates the suffix but may change the word (Brahmi et al., 2012). An example of this can be seen in Table 4.3 below.

Original Word	**Stemmed**	**Lemmatized**
Studying	Study	Study
Studied	Studi	Study

Table 4.2 – Example comparing stemming and lemmatization

Lemmatization is preferred when preserving context is necessary; however, it is contingent on a linguistic dictionary for the script to look up a specific root word. If the word's form is not included in the lemmatization dictionary, it may not be interpreted correctly and subsequently affect LDA results. Conversely, stemming is simpler to implement, but humans will spend more time analyzing the results. One would need to know that study and studi are referring to the same topic in the example. LDA could be run on the raw text, but there will be more words to interpret within the analysis without stemming or completing lemmatization. There is a risk-benefit trade when opting to stem or lemmatize the data. Most authors maintain using one of these methods is the best way to prepare data for LDA, and neither technique is superior (Blei et al., 2003; Jipeng, Zhenyu, Yun, Yunhao, & Xindong, 2019; Zuo, Zhao, & Xu, 2016).

Data Analysis

Although an older version of the MALLET distribution for LDA was used by Ranard et al. (2016), the package has not had updates since 2016. I opted to use the Gensim distribution due to ease of installation, increased reference material available to help with the analysis and regular updates. Anecdotal research by Akef, Munoz Arango, & Xu (2016) has indicated that MALLET and Gensim perform similar actions, but the outputs of word groupings can differ. While attempting to complete LDA analysis using Gensim, I encountered difficulties obtaining meaningful word groupings across topics, so I switched to an open-source javascript code that better handled short text. Samples of the raw output of using Gensim are included in Appendix D. I selected Word Network Topic Modelling (WNTM) LDA as this was found to have improvements over traditional LDA such as Gensim and MALLET (Zuo et al., 2016). Since the Ranard et al. (2016) study was completed several years ago, there have been gains about categorizing short text using LDA. Short text documents such as user reviews and other social media posts are described as having sparse data within each document, making it difficult to identify meaningful groups of words using standard LDA methods (Zuo et al., 2016). The most significant difference between methods is that WNTM assumes that each document consists of a single topic, whereas traditional LDA does not make that assumption. This assumption changes how words are mapped across each document, as the focus is on the frequency of words within each short text document, as opposed to the topics that emerge from long text documents (Zuo et al., 2016). The WNTM javascript program made by Zuo et al. (2016) is open source and readily available to use on github.com (Jipeng et al., 2019). Open source indicates that it may be freely used and modified as required, as long as the code is not used for profit (Red Hat Inc., 2020).

Similar to the Ranard et al. (2016) study, I ran the analysis using groupings of seven words for one to ten, 15, 20, 25, 50, 75, 100, 150 and 200 topics. However, my work differed from Ranard et al. (2016), as I also ran the analysis for smaller topic numbers to determine what the word groupings would reveal. The WNTM LDA model's hyperparameters were not modified from the default setting as these were already optimized for short text user reviews (Zuo et al., 2016). Coherence and perplexity scores were not calculated because the values did not aid human judgement in interpretation (Le, Weber, & Wild, 2020). One of my reasons for doing this was that my experience as a health care professional in various settings had provided me the context to interpret the findings. An assumption in the interpretation of my findings is that my experience in health care could bias the results. As I have some emergency and critical care experience this likely biased my interpretation of the LDA word groupings. Conversely as I have little ambulatory experience, themes related to this may have not been as prominent in my interpretation. As mentioned in Chapter 3, knowing the subject matter does affect and can aid the interpretation of results due to the loss of context.

Reflexive Thematic Analysis

Ranard et al. (2016) also did not use coherence and perplexity to determine the correct number of topics. Instead, the researchers interpreted topics by reading word groupings and assigning a topic name to each word grouping per series. Ranard et al. (2016) did not specify the methodology used to identify topics. I gave topic names to each word grouping using reflexive thematic analysis by Braun & Clarke (2006) to identify topics from the word groupings. Shovkun, Fleischmann, & Xie (2018) and Fleischmann et al., (2015) identified topics using Thematic Analysis by having multiple authors read the outputs of the LDA analysis. Reflexive Thematic Analysis is characterized by the active participation of the researcher in knowledge creation (Byrne, 2021). The codes or themes as identified by the researcher are patterns that have been interpreted through the review of the data. In using reflexive thematic analysis, it is not unexpected that themes or codes may be different across researchers examining the same data set(Byrne, 2021). The process by which the codes arise is organic and flexible. Themes are meant to change as familiarity with the data set increases. I used a combination of inductive and deductive reflexive thematic analysis as described in each of the analysis below. Each analysis was completed using Microsoft Excel. Microsoft Excel was selected as it was convenient to drag and drop cells containing topics, word groupings or codes under columns that contained topic names or survey measures and domains. Specifics of the use of Excel are contained within each analysis below.

Identifying the Correct Topics and Topic Number

I selected the topic number based on careful study of the word groupings across the various topic numbers. This first mapping of word groups to topic names used an inductive thematic analysis approach. Due to lack of context, I used my existing knowledge of healthcare to supplement the codes and themes that arose from the data. The word groupings were each put into a spreadsheet with a single tab that contained each cohort of word groupings. Each grouping was assigned a topic or code based on this my interpretation of the data. I gave the same topic name or code to that word grouping where I felt word groupings were similar. As I went through each topic number's word groupings if a code appeared that fit a grouping better, I went back to the previous topic numbers and re-coded the data to reflect the new topic across the data set. If the codes were dissimilar, a new code was created. The process was repeated across all topics until each word grouping within every topic number had a code. Similar codes were generated across all topic numbers; however, the 200 topics identified various topics compared to the analysis completed with the lower topic numbers. Thus 200 topics was selected as the correct number of topics. The identified topic names for the 200 topics is presented in table 5.1 of Chapter 5. The raw word groupings mapped to each topic name is given in Appendix E. Samples of the raw data from the other topic numbers are presented in Appendix F.

Mapping Topics to CPES-IC Measures

Once the correct number of topics was identified, topics were mapped to CPES-IC measures again using a reflexive thematic analysis approach through my interpretation of the relationship between identified topics and the CPES-IC measures. The topics were mapped to the CPES-IC measures in an excel spreadsheet. The topics from the 200 topic number analysis had duplicates removed so only unique topics remained. The remaining topics were then mapped in a single excel spreadsheet tab with each column indicating a separate CPES-IC measure. In this case, a deductive approach was taken to map the topic names to the CPES-IC measures. When there were no relatable measures, the raw data from the word groupings was reviewed and compared with the CPES-IC questions associated with each CPES-IC measure. Where the raw data provided additional context, those topics were mapped to the appropriate CPES-IC measure on the excel spreadsheet. Although topics names in the 'No Category' category may have been associated with a CPES-IC measure, there may have been insufficient context in the raw word groupings to determine association with the CPES-IC measures, according to my judgement. The topic name mapping to CPES-IC measure can be seen in Table 5.1 in Chapter 5. For a mapping of CPES-IC questions to CPES-IC measures, see Appendix G.

Newly Identified Topics from LDA Analysis

Topics that remained uncategorized after mapping the LDA topics to the CPES-IC measures were assigned to a measure that I identified using reflexive thematic analysis on the topics that emerged from the first analysis. Again, these were mapped in a single tab of an excel spreadsheet where the remaining LDA topics were examined and grouped together using deductive thematic analysis. I identified patterns across topics and grouped them together.

Validating the Effectiveness of the LDA Analysis

As this work's analysis using LDA differed from Ranard et al. (2016), a check for effectiveness was completed to ensure results were similar to the topics found by LDA. Of the total reviews downloaded, each review was assigned a random number and ordered from highest to lowest using excel. The first 100 reviews were selected to determine the number of contained topics within each. The same 100 reviews were also reviewed to determine if the LDA analysis topics were present in topics identified through manual coding. The table below provides descriptive statistics of the 100 review sample.

Total Reviews	Average Words	Median Words	Maximum Words	Minimum Words	Standard Deviation
100	63.92	38	275	2	60.87

Table 4.3 – Descriptive statistics for 100 randomly selected reviews for manual coding

Samples and results of this analysis are presented in Chapter 5. The raw data analysis is included in Appendix H. The manual coding was completed using thematic analysis. Each review was put into a single cell in an Excel spreadsheet. Topics that emerged from each review were put in the column beside. If a review had more than one topic present it was placed underneath the preceding topic in the topics column. If a review had similar codes, I would go back to previous reviews and determine if those codes should be changed or if the new code was novel.

Newly Identified Measures from Manually Coded Topics

The uncategorized topics were mapped similar to the LDA analysis for identifying new measures process above. Any remaining uncategorized topics were grouped under new measures.

Comparison to HCAHPs Domains and CPES-IC Domains

As the HCAHPS and CPES-IC domains contain fewer categories compared to the CPES-IC measures, the LDA topics were also mapped to determine if the topics found by the LDA analysis could be mapped to the fewer categories for the HCAHPS and CPES-IC, respectively. This analysis was carried out similarly to the LDA analysis using the CPES-IC Measures. The procedure remained the same, however the data the topics were mapped to differed.

Chapter 5 - Results

The results are reported in several tables. The first depicts all the topics identified using Latent Dirchlet Allocation (LDA) mapped to the CPES-IC measures. The following table lists topics that were not categorized were grouped under new measures that I identified. The next section is a check of the effectiveness of this LDA analysis that maps the LDA topics to the HCAHPS and CPES-IC domains. The last tables are from a manual coding analysis of topics from 100 reviews. The first table maps the manually coded topics to the CPES-IC measures, and the final table maps the uncategorized topics to the measures I identified using the LDA topics, including measures that were only identified in the manual coding data.

Mapping to CPES-IC Measures

LDA topics were mapped to the measures in the CPES-IC (Table 5.1). Topics that were not mapped to a category were categorized under No Category. CPES-IC categories that were not assigned topics are indicated by the statement 'no topics mapped.' These include: 'Transfer from ED to Hospital Bed Organized', 'Admission to Hospital Organized', 'Discharge Planning', 'Discharge Management', and 'Internal Coordination of Care'.

dmission through ED	All Hospital Admissions	No Category
Waiting too Long in the ED for a Hospital Bed	**Cleanliness**	Ambulation
Emergency Wait time	Cleanliness of Physical Environment	Appreciation for Staff
Wait Time and Waiting Room	**Communication with Doctors**	Assessment
Information Shared with Patients in the Emergency	Physician Care	Busy emergency room
Emergency Room Care	Physician Communication	Care of Family Member
Transfer from ED to Hospital Bed Organized	Physician Written Communication	Communication
o Topics Mapped)	**Communication with Nurses**	Comparing Hospital Care
rect Admission	Likeability of Nursing Staff	Comparing hospital to walk in clinic
ough Information Given about Admission Process Prior to Arrival	**Coordination of Tests and Procedures**	Comparison of Emergency to Walk-In Clinic
(No Topics Mapped)	Diagnostic Tests	Comparison of Emergency Visits
dmission to Hospital Organized	Wait for Lab Test	Comparison of Hospital Emergency Rooms
(No Topics Mapped)	**Discharge Planning**	Dressing Change
	(No Topics Mapped)	Emergency Cardiac Care
	Discharge Management	Emergency Care
	(No Topics Mapped)	Emergency Staff Attitude
	Emotional Support	Experience over the Phone
	Mental Comfort	Feelings about Care
	Rude Staff	Getting to the Hospital
	Thoughts about treatment	Healthcare System
	Explanation about Medications	Hospital Comparison
	Immunization	Hospital Food
	Medication Side Effects	Intravenous Experience
	Prescription	Lab Test Experience
	Hospital Rating (Worst to Best)	Length of Hospital Stay
	Overall Rating	Male Nurse Care
	Hospital Stay Helpful	Maternity Care
	No Topics Mapped	Mental Health Care
	Intent to Recommend Hospital to Family and Friends	Motor Vehicle Accident Care
	Recommend to Others	Multiple Visits for Same Issue
	Reviewing Experience of Care for Others	Nighttime Checks
	Involvement in Decision-Making	No Phone for Use
	Communication about surgery	Nursing Attitude
	Communication to Family and Friends	Nursing Unit Care
	Family Care	Parking
	Internal Coordination of Care	Pediatric Care
	(No Topics Mapped)	Physical and Mental Environment
	Overall Hospital Experience (Very Poor to Very Good)	Physical Building
	Overall Experience	Physical Comfort
	Quality of Care	Physical Safety
	Pain Controlled	Physician Emergency Care
	Medication for Pain Control	Physiotherapist Care
	Pain Control	Previous Experience of Care
	Pain Control during Procedure	Quality vs Value
	Pain Control for Family	Referral to Another Department
	Wait Time for Pain Control	Respiratory Care
	Quietness	Seeking Healthcare
	Physical Environment	Social Worker Care
	Received Information about Condition and Treatment	Staff Attitude
	Oncology Care	Staff Care
	Recognition of Health Issue	Staff Communication
	Treatment	Staff Gender
	Unclear instructions	Staff Workload
	Staff Responsiveness	Student Nurse Care
	Help when Needed	Surgical Care
	Request to see Staff	Tax Dollars on Healthcare
	Waiting for Doctor	Thoughts about Staff
		Timeframe of Experience
		Transfer between Hospitals
		University Affiliated Hospitals
		Wait Time
		Wait Time Comparison between Hospitals
		Wait time for Appointment
		Wait Time for Subjective Severity of Health Issue
		Waiting for Emergency Physician
		Waiting for Physician
		Waiting for results
		Waiting for Staff
		Waiting for Treatment
		Waiting Room Experience
		Wayfinding
		Wound Dressing

ble 5.1 – LDA Topics to CPES-IC Measures Mapping

Table 5.2 below lists the unmapped LDA topics from Table 5.1 mapped to new measures that emerged from the LDA topics. Seventeen new measures were identified, and all remaining topics were mapped to these measures.

Allied Healthcare	**Healthcare System**
Physiotherapist Care	Healthcare System
Social Worker Care	Quality vs. Value
Area or Type of Care	Tax Dollars on Healthcare
Emergency Cardiac Care	**Hospital Stay**
Emergency Care	Length of Hospital Stay
Emergency Room Care	No Phone for Use
Maternity Care	Timeframe of Experience
Mental Comfort	**Overall Staff Rating**
Mental Health Care	Thoughts about Staff
MVA Care	**Parking**
Nursing Unit Care	Parking
Oncology Care	**Physical Environment**
Pediatric Care	Physical Building
Respiratory Care	Physical Comfort
Surgical Care	Physical Environment
University Affiliated Hospitals	**Staff Availability**
Before Receiving Care	Busy emergency room
Getting to the Hospital	Staff Workload
Seeking Healthcare	**Student Care**
Wayfinding	Student Nurse Care
Being Thankful to have Healthcare	**Treatment Experience**
Appreciation for Staff	Ambulation
Care of Family Member	Assessment
Care of Family Member	Dressing Change
Comparing Healthcare Services	Intravenous Experience
Comparing Hospital Care	Nighttime Checks
Comparing hospital to walk-in clinic	Recognition of Health Issue
Comparison of emergency to walk-in clinic	Treatment
Comparison of emergency visits	Wound Dressing
Comparison of Hospital Emergency Rooms	**Wait Time**
Hospital Comparison	Wait for Lab Test
Previous Experience of Care	Wait Time and Waiting Room
Wait Time Comparison between Hospitals	Wait time for Appointment
Food	Waiting for Emergency Physician
Hospital Food	Waiting for Treatment
Gender of Staff	Waiting Room Experience
Male Nurse Care	
Staff Gender	

Table 5.2 – Additional Measures Identified from the Non-Categorized LDA Topics

Mapping to the HCAHPS Domains

LDA obtained topics were mapped to the HCAHPS domains to determine if the use of measures changed the ability to map topics (Table 5.3). Of the ten domains in the HCAHPS survey, all had topics that were mapped. Of the 109 topics, 73 were unmapped to the HCAHPS domains.

Cleanliness of Hospital Environment	**No Category**	**No Category**
Cleanliness of Physical Environment	Ambulation	Quality of Care
Communication about medications	Appreciation for Staff	Quality vs Value
Immunization	Assessment	Recognition of Health Issue
Medication Side Effects	Busy emergency room	Respiratory Care
Prescription	Care of Family Member	Seeking Healthcare
Communication with doctors	Communication	Social Worker Care
Physician Care	Communication about surgery	Staff Gender
Physician Communication	Communication to Family and Friends	Staff Workload
Physician Emergency Care	Comparing Hospital Care	Student Nurse Care
Physician Written Communication	Comparing hospital to walk in clinic	Surgical Care
Communication with nurses	Comparison of Emergency to Walk In Clinic	Tax Dollars on Healthcare
Likeability of Nursing Staff	Comparison of Emergency Visits	Thoughts about Staff
Nursing Attitude	Comparison of Hospital Emergency Rooms	Thoughts about treatment
Discharge information	Diagnostic Tests	Timeframe of Experience
Multiple Visits for Same Issue	Dressing Change	Transfer between Hospitals
Referral to Another Department	Emergency Cardiac Care	Treatment
Global hospital experience - Hospital rating	Emergency Care	Unclear instructions
Overall Experience	Emergency Room Care	University Affiliated Hospitals
Overall Rating	Experience over the Phone	Wait for Lab Test
Global hospital experience - Will Recommend Hospital	Family Care	Wait Time and Waiting Room
Recommend to Others	Feelings about Care	Wait Time Comparison between Hospitals
Reviewing Experience of Care for Others	Getting to the Hospital	Wait time for Appointment
Pain control	Healthcare System	Wait Time for Subjective Severity of Health Issue
Medication for Pain Control	Hospital Comparison	Waiting for results
Pain Control	Hospital Food	Waiting for Treatment
Pain Control during Procedure	Intravenous Experience	Waiting Room Experience
Pain Control for Family	Lab Test Experience	Wayfinding
Wait for Pain Control	Length of Hospital Stay	Wound Dressing
Wait Time for Pain Control	Male Nurse Care	
Quietness of Hospital Environment	Maternity Care	
Physical and Mental Environment	Mental Comfort	
Responsiveness of staff	Mental Health Care	
Emergency Staff Attitude	MVA Care	
Emergency Wait time	Nighttime Checks	
Help when Needed	No Phone for Use	
Request to see Staff	Nursing Unit Care	
Rude Staff	Oncology Care	
Staff Attitude	Parking	
Staff Care	Pediatric Care	
Staff Communication	Physical Building	
Wait Time	Physical Comfort	
Waiting for Doctor	Physical Environment	
Waiting for Emergency Physician	Physical Safety	
Waiting for Physician	Physiotherapist Care	
Waiting for Staff	Previous Experience of Care	

Table 5.3 – LDA identified topics mapped to HCAHPS domains

Mapping to CPES-IC Domains

Table 5.4 is a mapping of the LDA obtained topics to the CPES-IC domains to determine if mapping to fewer topics would improve the mapping. Of the 109 topics, 59 were not mapped to any of the CPES-IC domains. Of the 22 domains identified in the CPES-IC, only 21 were relevant to the analysis. Five CPES-IC domains did not have any LDA topics assigned: Admission through emergency department, Demographics, Direct Admit, Discharge information and Helped by hospital stay.

Admit through emergency department
- (No Topics Mapped)

Cleanliness of Hospital Environment
- Cleanliness of Physical Environment

Communication
- Communication
- Communication about surgery
- Experience over the Phone
- Rude Staff
- Staff Communication

Communication about medications
- Immunization
- Medication Side Effects
- Prescription

Communication with doctors
- Physician Care
- Physician Communication
- Physician Emergency Care
- Physician Written Communication

Communication with nurses
- Likeability of Nursing Staff
- Nursing Attitude

Demographic
- (No Topics Mapped)

Direct Admit
- (No Topics Mapped)

Discharge and transition
- Multiple Visits for Same Issue
- Transfer between Hospitals

Discharge Information
- (No Topics Mapped)

Emotional support
- Feelings about Care
- Staff Attitude

Global hospital experience - Hospital rating
- Overall Rating

Global hospital experience - Will Recommend Hospital
- Recommend to Others
- Reviewing Experience of Care for Others

Helped by Hospital Stay
- (No Topics Mapped)

Internal coordination of care
- Referral to Another Department

Involvement in decision-making
- Communication to Family and Friends
- Family Care
- Thoughts about treatment
- Unclear instructions

Outcome
- Quality of Care

Overall hospital experience
- Overall Experience

Pain control
- Medication for Pain Control
- Pain Control
- Pain Control during Procedure
- Pain Control for Family
- Wait for Pain Control
- Wait Time for Pain Control

Patient Safety
- Physical Safety

Quietness of Hospital Environment
- Physical and Mental Environment

Responsiveness of staff
- Emergency Staff Attitude
- Emergency Wait time
- Help when Needed
- Request to see Staff
- Staff Care
- Wait Time
- Wait Time for Subjective Severity of Health Issue
- Waiting for Doctor
- Waiting for Physician
- Waiting for Staff

Timeliness of testing
- Diagnostic Tests
- Lab Test Experience
- Waiting for results

No Category
- Ambulation
- Appreciation for Staff
- Assessment
- Busy emergency room
- Care of Family Member
- Comparing Hospital Care
- Comparing hospital to walk in clinic
- Comparison of Emergency to Walk In Clinic
- Comparison of Emergency Visits
- Comparison of Hospital Emergency Rooms
- Dressing Change
- Emergency Cardiac Care
- Emergency Care
- Emergency Room Care
- Getting to the Hospital
- Healthcare System
- Hospital Comparison

No Category (continued)
- Hospital Food
- Intravenous Experience
- Length of Hospital Stay
- Male Nurse Care
- Maternity Care
- Mental Comfort
- Mental Health Care
- MVA Care
- Nighttime Checks
- No Phone for Use
- Nursing Unit Care
- Oncology Care
- Parking
- Pediatric Care
- Physical Building
- Physical Comfort
- Physical Environment
- Physiotherapist Care
- Previous Experience of Care
- Quality vs Value
- Recognition of Health Issue
- Respiratory Care
- Seeking Healthcare
- Social Worker Care
- Staff Gender
- Staff Workload
- Student Nurse Care
- Surgical Care
- Tax Dollars on Healthcare
- Thoughts about Staff
- Timeframe of Experience
- Treatment
- University Affiliated Hospitals
- Wait for Lab Test
- Wait Time and Waiting Room
- Wait Time Comparison between Hospitals
- Wait time for Appointment
- Waiting for Emergency Physician
- Waiting for Treatment
- Waiting Room Experience
- Wayfinding
- Wound Dressing

Table 5.4 – LDA Identified topics mapped to CPES-IC domains

Effectiveness of LDA with CPES-IC Measures

Table 5.5 is a mapping of topics obtained through manual coding of 100 reviews to the CPES-IC measures as a method of evaluating the effectiveness of LDA. In the manual process, initially, 261 topics were identified, which resulted in 129 unique topics. Of the twenty-three CPES-IC measures, six did not have topics including: Information shared with patients in the emergency, transfer from ED to Hospital Bed Organized, Enough information given about admission process prior to arrival, admission to hospital organized, discharge planning, and internal coordination of care. Of the 129 unique topics, 77 were not mapped to any of the CPES-IC measures.

Admission through ED	All Hospital Admissions	No Category
Waiting too Long in the ED for a Hospital Bed	**Cleanliness**	1st experience
Emergency Wait Time	Cleanliness of Bathroom	Ambulatory care
Information Shared with Patients in the Emergency	Cleanliness of Physical Environment	Appointment Wait Time
(No Topics Mapped)	**Communication with Doctors**	Aspiration
Transfer from ED to Hospital Bed Organized	Busy Doctor	Bad experience
(No Topics Mapped)	Emergency Physician Care	Broken Bones
Direct Admission	Physician Attitude	Broken Hand
Enough Information Given about Admission Process Prior to Arrival	Physician Care	Cancer
(No Topics Mapped)	Surgeon Attitude	Car Accidents
Admission to Hospital Organized	**Communication with Nurses**	Cardiac Care
(No Topics Mapped)	Emergency Nurse Care	Cast
	Nurse Attitude	Chairs in the Waiting Room
	Coordination of Tests and Procedures	Comparison to other hospitals
	Diagnostic Test	Comparison to a Monkey
	Imaging Wait Time	Comparison to a veterinarian
	Discharge Planning	Comparison to family doctor
	(No Topics Mapped)	Comparison to Walk in Clinic
	Discharge Management	Comparison vs private health care
	Early discharge	Cost of Service
	Emotional Support	Date of care
	Felt not understood	Day Surgery
	Explanation about Medications	Deaths in Hospital
	Medication Instructions	Difficulty finding staff
	Hospital Rating (Worst to Best)	Donating to Hospital
	Overall Hospital Rating	Emergency Admitting
	Hospital Stay Helpful	Emergency Department Care
	Thankful for Care	Health Condition
	Intent to Recommend Hospital to Family and Friends	Hysteroscopy
	Recommend Hospital to Others	Intravenous Insertion Experience
	Recommend Others to go to this Hospital	IV Treatment
	Would have procedure again	Knee injury
	Would not recommend hospital	Lack of Care
	Would Visit Hospital Again	Lack of Pediatrician
	Involvement in Decision-Making	Lack of Surgeons
	Asking for help for a loved one	Length of Stay
	Care of Loved One	Long Weekend
	Forced treatment	Looking for Work
	Overnight Stay Policy	Male Nurse Care
	Internal Coordination of Care	Management Attitude
	(No Topics Mapped)	Management does not care
	Overall Hospital Experience (Very Poor to Very Good)	Maternity Care
	Experience of Care	Misdiagnosis
	Pain Controlled	Missed lunch
	Pain Control	Missed Medication
	Quietness	N/A
	Physical environment	Nurses Sleep on Nightshift
	Received Information about Condition and Treatment	Nursing care
	Felt Informed	Overall Staff Rating
	Waiting for Diagnosis	Palliative Care
	Staff Responsiveness	Parking Cost
	Excellent staff care	Parking Issues
	Experience of One Staff Member	Parking Lot Staff
		Permanent damage from care
		Physical Building
		Quality Improvement
		Quality of Food
		Response to other reviews
		Rural Hospital Closure
		Short staffed
		Signage
		Social Distancing
		Staff Attitude
		Staff attractiveness
		Staff Care
		Subsequent Visit
		Surgical care
		Surgical Experience
		Time of care
		Treatment
		Treatment by Staff
		Treatment of other Patients
		Triage Nurse Training
		Visiting Hours
		Volunteer care
		Wait time
		Went to another hospital
		Women's Health

Table 5.5 – 100 Manually Analyzed Review Topics mapped to CPES-IC measures

Table 5.6 lists the unmapped topics from the manual analysis of 100 reviews in Table 5.5. These unmapped topics were mapped to the new measures identified in Table 5.2. Of the 17 measures identified in the LDA analysis, five did not have topics mapped. This table also includes 11 new measures that were not identified in the LDA analysis but emerged from the manual data analysis.

Allied Healthcare	**Comparing Healthcare Services**	**Staff Availability**	**New Measures from Manual Analysis**
(No Topics Mapped)	Comparison to a Monkey	Difficulty finding staff	**COVID-19**
Area or Type of Care	Comparison to a veterinarian	Lack of Care	Social Distancing
Ambulatory care	Comparison to family doctor	Lack of Pediatrician	**Donations**
Aspiration	Comparison to other hospitals	Lack of Surgeons	Donating to Hospital
Broken Bones	Comparison to Walk in Clinic	Nurses Sleep on Nightshift	**Hospital Management**
Broken Hand	Comparison vs private health care	Short staffed	Management Attitude
Cancer	**Food**	**Student Care**	Management does not care
Car Accidents	Missed lunch	(No Topics Mapped)	**Job Seeking**
Cardiac Care	Quality of Food	**Treatment Experience**	Looking for Work
Cast	**Gender of Staff**	1st experience	**Quality Improvement**
Day Surgery	Male Nurse Care	Bad experience	Quality Improvement
Emergency Admitting	**Healthcare System**	Deaths in Hospital	**Related to other Reviews**
Emergency Department Care	Cost of Service	Intravenous Insertion Experience	Response to other reviews
Health Condition	**Hospital Stay**	Misdiagnosis	**Rural Care**
Hysteroscopy	Length of Stay	Missed Medication	Rural Hospital Closure
IV Treatment	Long Weekend	Permanent damage from care	**Staff Attractiveness**
Knee injury	Visiting Hours	Staff Attitude	Staff attractiveness
Maternity Care	**Overall Staff Rating**	Staff Care	**Staff Training**
Nursing care	Overall Staff Rating	Treatment	Triage Nurse Training
Palliative Care	**Parking**	Treatment by Staff	**Time/Date**
Subsequent Visit	Parking Cost	Treatment of other Patients	Date of care
Surgical care	Parking Issues	**Wait Time**	Time of care
Surgical Experience	Parking Lot Staff	Appointment Wait Time	**Volunteer Care**
Women's Health	**Physical Environment**	Wait time	Volunteer care
Before Receiving Care	Chairs in the Waiting Room	Went to another hospital	
(No Topics Mapped)	Physical Building		
Being Thankful to have Healthcare	Signage		
(No Topics Mapped)			
Care of Family Member			
(No Topics Mapped)			

Table 5.6 – Manually coded topics mapped to additional domains from LDA analysis plus new domains from manual analysis.

Chapter 6 – Discussion

Introduction

The results provide evidence that free-text Google user reviews of acute care hospitals in BC contain information relevant to the CPES-IC measures. There is also evidence that the same free-text user reviews contain information not included in the measures of the CPES-IC. As a measure of hospital processes, the patient experience captured in free-text user reviews has information tracked by the CPES-IC and information important to patients.

The current iteration of the CPES-IC created a national survey to benchmark services for quality improvement using patient experience. The CPES-IC is still relatively new, except for the HCAHP questions. Each measure's purpose has not yet been identified save for the ability to benchmark scores across jurisdictions and services.

Not every CPES-IC measure was represented within this work's analysis. This may have been related to methodology or inclusion of topics that policy-makers and administrators determined were important, which may be less relevant to the population of patients and families writing free-text reviews. This chapter will discuss these findings, future investigations, nursing and health informatics implications, and limitations.

Significant Findings

Similarity to Previous Work

Ranard et al. (2016) were able to find topics in Yelp user reviews for each domain within the HCAHPS, and each HCAHPS domain was represented by topics in the Google User Reviews in this study (Table 5.3). This adds to evidence that online free text user reviews contain information captured in the HCAHPS domains and that this finding may hold in the Canadian context.

Usefulness in the Canadian Context

Not all domains of the CPES-IC were found in British Columbia hospital Google reviews. The CPES-IC stratifies the domains into 23 measures rather than the HCAHPS' ten. The additional thirteen measures in the Canadian survey may have contributed to the inability to find topics using LDA. Further stratifying the original domains has increased the specificity of the survey, which may have caused the algorithm or my interpretation of the algorithim not to find relevant topics.

The CPES-IC measures examine specific information relevant to the patient's experience. You may recall in Chapter 2 of this work; the CPES-IC is a patient experience survey focused on health system accountability (Hadibhai et al., 2018). It is also essential to remember that Larson et al. (2019) suggest that individual patient experience measures can be focused on evaluating health system accountability or providing quality care but not both simultaneously. Google users may not have written about the missing CPES-IC measures; however, users may be less concerned about overall health system accountability and instead focused on the processes of care which are important to them.

Of the 23 measures in the CPES-IC, six contained no topics from the Latent Dirichlet Allocation (LDA) analysis of the Google user reviews. Most of these measures were related to the subjects of discharge or admission. This finding is consistent with manually coded topics from the 100 randomly selected reviews. LDA and manual analysis differed in two categories: information shared with patients in the emergency department; and discharge management. These differences might be attributed to the data from the manually coded sample, type of LDA analysis completed, bias in the thematic analysis of mapping word groupings to topic names or bias during mapping topics to CPES-IC measures. These discrepancies could have happened in both the LDA data thematic analysis and the thematic analysis for manually coded data. The significant difference between the two analyses is that the LDA analysis was conducted on groupings of words without additional context. In contrast, the manually coded data was obtained from reading individual reviews, which provided context. The analytic process difference likely contributed to the difference in CPES-IC measures identified. As discussed in Chapter 3, LDA analysis is often 80% accurate in categorizing data correctly, and data might be missing due to the LDA analysis (Roitblat, 2020). As LDA analysis is sensitive to the pre-identified topic number, the number of topics selected may not have been sufficient to capture the difference. However, the LDA analysis only examined word groupings up to 200 topics in this work. Higher topic numbers could have included additional CPES-IC measures, however as the topic number increases, the time to analyze the data also increases.

Although not the focus of this work, while patient satisfaction is an outcome of the experience of care, it is essential to recall that motivation for writing a review may be based on satisfaction (Lantzy, Hamilton, Chen, & Stewart, 2020). Whether or not an evidence-based interaction occurred may matter less to the patient, which could have caused users to omit those events when writing their reviews (Lantzy et al., 2020; Larson et al., 2019). This does not challenge the legitimacy of a user's review; a consumer may omit information that is of interest to health care professionals and administrators for reasons such as lack of interest in writing a review about it (Lantzy et al., 2020). It is feasible that health care consumers may have experienced these events, but they may not be motivated to write as frequently about these events. Concerning the missing measures, it may be that users writing reviews did not feel the process of admission or discharge was worth noting, even though this is a focus in health care (Leamy, Thompson, & Mitra, 2019).

Possible Differences with Previous Work

A second explanation for missing topics is that the LDA I used to categorize the user reviews could have affected the results. While Ranard et al. (2016) used LDA included in the Machine Learning for Language Toolkit (MALLET) to determine word groupings from the Yelp user reviews, I employed word network topic modelling (WNTM) to obtain word groupings. A major difference in the assumptions between MALLET and WNTM is that WNTM assumes that the collection of documents is less critical than the words that co-occur within each document. In contrast, traditional LDA such as MALLET looks for co-occurring topics within all documents as a whole. It has also been demonstrated that traditional LDA methods such as MALLET do not handle short text documents as well as WNTM (Zuo et al., 2016). Although analysis was not completed using MALLET LDA compared with WNTM LDA, the manual coding analysis (Table 5.5) demonstrates shared topics and similar mapping to measures compared with the WNTM LDA analysis.

Given that many Google user reviews obtained in this work were short in length, the impact of having used WNTM as opposed to MALLET is unknown. This may be an avenue for future research; however, the research is clear that results are superior using

WNTM compared with traditional LDA (Zuo et al., 2016). While differences in methodology between Ranard et al. (2016) may have been another contributing factor for the missing topics, other differences during the data preparation step may have led to this result.

As mentioned in Chapter 3 on LDA, data preparation and cleaning are critical steps to perform before running LDA. Other than the high-level steps described by Ranard et al. (2016), it is unknown what exact steps were used to clean their Yelp review data. I propose two areas that may have differed: (1) instead of stemming the data, lemmatization was used; and (2) there were differences in which stop words were removed. For a review on the concepts of stemming and lemmatization, please see Chapter 4. While word stemming and lemmatization are similar in that these linguistic techniques transform words into a format that is easier to process, there are key differences (Brahmi et al., 2012). Stemming a word removes suffixes but does not transform words, where lemmatization not only removes the suffix but may change the word (Brahmi et al., 2012). In this analysis, I could not determine if the linguistic dictionary used to lemmatize the data contained all forms of words to ensure the same root word was found each time which may have affected the results of the analysis. However, it is outside the scope to discuss the lemmatizer's linguistic interpretation in this analysis.

Stop word removal may have also contributed to the missing topics, as I used the dictionary for stop words included with Natural Language Toolkit (NLTK). For additional information about stop words, please see Chapter 3 on LDA. Ranard et al. (2016) may have used the MALLET stop words dictionary, which has had less frequent updates than the NLTK stop words used in this work (Bird, Loper, & Klein, 2009; McCallum, 2002). Stop words typically indicate words that do not provide LDA context; however, stop words are subject matter dependent (HaCohen-Kerner, Miller, & Yigal, 2020). It is possible that stop word differences in other subject matter removed words that may have been beneficial to analyzing hospital reviews. HaCohen-Kerner et al. (2020) have found that removing stop words can have detrimental and advantageous effects on LDA results. In some instances, stop word removal should not be completed. HaCohen-Kerner et al. (2020) suggest experimenting with the data set before proceeding with LDA. However, this LDA analysis did not experiment without removing stop words, as the best procedure at the time of the analysis indicated that stop word removal was essential.

Topics Not Found in the CPES-IC

Of the list of topics in Table 5.1, 73 were not categorized in the CPES-IC measures. Although some of these may be attributed to methodology issues similar to the previous section, this may prove that Google user reviews contain topics not found in the CPES-IC categories. This would indicate that health care consumers care about health care topics that the CPES-IC does not address.

Several other explanations could have contributed to the uncategorized LDA topics. Given that I mapped word groupings to topics and subsequently topics to CPES-IC categories, there might have been bias introduced during both mappings. The use of reflexive thematic analysis provided an approach for recognizing and addressing bias (Braun & Clarke, 2006). What made this analysis challenging was using both an inductive approach when coding word groupings into topics and then using a deductive approach when coding the topics into measures. Without obtaining additional context from reading each review, it was difficult to code this data without the two different approaches. For example, when mapping LDA topics to CPES-IC categories 'emergency staff attitude', I opted to have this remain uncategorized even though it may have been possible to fit within the CPES-IC categories of Communication with Doctors and Communication with Nurses. Taking this example further, the words within the 'emergency staff attitude' topic could have also been mapped to the 'staff attitude' topic. However, I interpreted the words in the 'emergency staff attitude' topic as separate, as in this example, the word 'emergency' was present. However, it is important to note that my personal and professional experiences in health care may have contributed to the topic names, mapping to measures and new measures identified in this analysis.

During the manual coding analysis of the 100 reviews, it is important to note that similar topics arose in the data. However, the previous LDA analysis may have influenced those topic names. This may prove that the LDA topics are correct, but my perspective may also have been changed during the two analyses. An example of this might be demonstrated with the CPES-IC 'overall hospital rating' measure. In the LDA analysis, there were two topics related to this measure: quality and overall experience. With the manual analysis, when reading the reviews, I coded many topics under this single topic as I determined that many statements in reviews related to the overall hospital rating. This may have been a result of seeing the LDA word groupings first. Had I not completed the LDA analysis first, these multiple statements may have been categorized differently.

Future Areas for Research

This research has demonstrated proof of concept that online free-text user reviews include information that is contained within the categories and information outside of the categories of the CPES-IC. Like the Ranard et al. (2016) study, this work may prove that free-text user reviews can supplement traditional survey methods. However, some areas require further exploration to utilize this approach in practice. One important area to explore is determining what information contained within the reviews could actually be used by staff, operations leadership and executives to guide or improve patient-centred care. Initial exploration in this area has determined that free-text review validity might depend on the context (McGrath, Priestley, Zhou, & Culligan, 2018). Not all reviews may be helpful, and not all parts of an individual review might be useful. Determining the context or what parts of a review have utility is important as the volume of user reviews may make it difficult to read through each review. While natural language processing methods could help with this, it would still be difficult to analyze a large dataset without a sufficient understanding of what a human should be looking for.

It is well known what aspects of patient-centred care have been demonstrated to improve patient outcomes (Frampton et al., 2008). However, what is unknown is what aspects of patient-centred care can be gleaned from online social media free-text user reviews. Little research has been completed in this area in the literature. While patient-centred care information has been found in free-text comments from a traditional survey, this has not been extended to social media reviews (Ricci-Cabello, Saletti-Cuesta, Slight, & Valderas, 2017). Ricci-Cabello et al. (2017) suggest finding information related to patient-centred care in free-text reviews as these authors correlated the free-text responses from traditional surveys to the related questions from the survey. It is feasible that this could be extended to online free-text reviews connecting these to the CPES-IC questions.

A third area of research is exploring the use of LDA with respect to analyzing free-text user reviews in health care. Although additional literature has since been published since the Ranard et al. (2016) paper, there remain no best practices that can be easily leveraged for health organizations to employ (De Groof & Xu, 2017; Kowalski, 2017). The Nelson[5] (2020) method does hold some promise in this regard but would need additional research to determine how this could work using free-text user reviews for health care. Given the lack of standards and frameworks available to use LDA, determining the best way to implement LDA to categorize topics and analyze emerging trends in health care reviews is important. LDA is potentially a low-cost way to obtain quality improvement data (Rathore et al., 2016; Rose & Lennerholt, 2017). While LDA originally began in computer science, mathematics and linguistics, it is increasingly used in the social sciences (Nelson, 2020). Nelson (2020) has developed a methodological framework for natural language processing and qualitative analysis. Computational grounded theory[6] shows promise. It provides a rigorous framework to complete an analysis similar to this one by combining the best elements of computer and human interaction in a three-step methodology (Nelson, 2020). This methodology was not attempted as part of this work, although it might be worth exploring as it provides a framework and best practices to complete this type of research.

---

[5] The Nelson method refers to computational grounded theory. See Nelson (2020) for additional information

[6] Computational grounded theory is a methodological framework to integrate elements of human and computer interaction using grounded theory. See Nelson (2020) for additional information.

Implications for Nursing

This research highlights two important areas for nursing practice: (1) to improve the understanding of the impact of technology on the nursing profession; and (2) to improve the understanding of how to implement technology like this within nursing. Nurses must understand the impact of these technologies on the work of nursing (Canadian Nurses Association & Canadian Nursing Informatics Association, 2017). While we are not utilizing analysis of free-text reviews in Canadian health care, it may be possible to see changes to standards of care, practice and policy reflected in a patient's experience in near time should we begin to use these. For example, there is potential to implement a change to a rotation that improves workload and observe if the patterns in patient experience data change over several reviews. "Rude staff" and "appreciation for staff" were topics that emerged from the user reviews. While these may be unrelated to patient-centred care, there may be an eventual link to patient-centred care. Workload may have contributed to those patients' reviews. Without additional qualifiers, it may be easy to attribute either event to the attitudes of staff themselves instead of system factors that may affect the patients' experiences.

By leveraging online review data to examine trends over time, quality improvement projects could see results in near time and longitudinally. Utilizing technology in this way could significantly enhance nursing practice. However, nursing practice and the systems within nurses practice are not generally implementing these technologies in Canada (Peltonen et al., 2019). Although entry-level and executive-level informatics competencies are being implemented, clear guidelines and pathways are lacking to incorporate these technologies in practice. The main suggestion is for nurses to continue to engage in additional training to determine the best ways to align technology and desired patient outcomes (Peltonen et al., 2019). A multipronged approach to educate nurses on the use of technology and decrease the system barriers is needed to encourage nursing to utilize this technology. This includes increasing the amount of graduate and doctoral prepared nurses in health information science and technology (Peltonen et al., 2019). Improving education of nurses is insufficient alone. Structures and systems need to be put into place to allow nurses to define how technology should be used to care for and interact with patients (Peltonen et al., 2019). While it may still take a number of years to see this technology in practice, simple steps to add infrastructure may be what's required in the short term. For example, providing sufficient computers for staff use, as using basic computer technology for home and community care is needed. It has been demonstrated that improving speed of a computer system greatly improves adoption, as a slow response time usually adds to user frustration (Strudwick, Hall, Nagle, & Trbovich, 2018). Improving speed is not something a point of care nurse is able to do and likely requires intervention from both management and technology support.

Additionally, from a nursing management perspective, health systems that allow for technology like LDA need to be developed. Currently, health jurisdictions do not have mechanisms to make and evaluate significant changes in near time that would not cause added stress to individuals. Continuing to develop roles that include nurse informaticists at the point of care is important as nurses with added informatics competencies understand clinical and technical environments (Thomas, Seifert, & Joyner, 2016). They are vital in integrating workflow changes that are less disruptive as they understand what it takes to implement a change due to technology. Not only would they be familiar with nurses' work, but they are also in a position to understand how to mitigate the impacts to work and determine if the technology is beneficial or harmful. Combined with well-developed unit-based or organizational key performance indicators, using a nurse informaticist to help improve KPIs through technology may be an excellent strategy to optimize existing or develop new workflows (Thomas et al., 2016).

This work is essential to nurses as nurses need to understand how technology like LDA works. Although it is not an individual nurse's responsibility is to understand every facet of technology that can improve patient care, it remains vital for nurses to know how the technology works and the rationale for use (Besworth, 2016). If we do not take advantage of emerging technologies, we can be left behind with innovations as other groups may quickly define how technology should be used for nursing (Huston, 2013). This is particularly important as nurses are the largest healthcare workforce closest to the point of care. Nurses are in a position to understand and address quality of care issues while focusing on improving patient-centred care.

Similarly, while this technology has the potential to help, it also has the potential to harm (Huston, 2013). Examining results without understanding how the methodology works may make this practice susceptible to Campbell's law, where the technology is leveraged only to improve a metric rather than improve patient care (Campbell, 1979). It is also important to note that technology and metrics should not be the underlying focus of nursing. Instead, the patient should be the focus and the centre of care. Technology is a tool and, if not correctly understood, could be implemented to introduce bias. For example, if you assume that user reviews from Google are representative of the population as a whole, that assumption may be incorrect. Only acting on data contained within the user reviews may cause you to make changes that may not entirely reflect the population as a whole. Understanding the technology and developing processes to ensure harm is not being introduced while utilizing this technology is just as important as leveraging the technology itself. Having nurses who use the technology and develop it are important pieces of a profession's ability to self-regulate (Canadian Nurses Association, 2015).

Implications for Health Informatics

This work highlights several uses of information technology to aid in data collection, retrieval and processing for health informaticians. Although not highlighted in this work, the modification of a python script to automatically download Google user reviews can make data collection more efficient. While this methodology is not unique nor novel to this work, reducing the time required to gather data improves the ability to analyze the data. Particularly once a script is written until the source website updates its coding, the script can continue to download user reviews for analysis with little intervention, but a button click from a user. With additional modification, the entire process could be automated; however, more development work would be required to achieve this. Saving time decreases the cost, allowing for the allocation of resources to other endeavors.

A second implication is that this work utilizes qualitative methods and combines these with computer processing to receive results in a shorter time frame while achieving accuracy levels that are 80% or greater. As evidenced by the results, there were many overlapping topics identified by both the LDA and manual coding analyses. This work adds additional credence to qualitative research methods that leverage computers to do manual processing. While research is still occurring in automated topic identification via LDA, it may be possible to train the computers to code data as a human would through more advanced methods.

Limitations of Study Methodology

Although there is promise to have natural language processing categorize user reviews automatically and detect both emerging and recurring themes in user reviews, there are limitations to the applicability of this technology and research for populations within healthcare. One of the most significant limitations to this type of technology is the barrier for those who do not have online access to write reviews (Bailey et al., 2015). While access to a computer or mobile device has been increasing, there remain members of the Canadian population who do not own a computer, use a mobile device, have internet access or have enough technology literacy to be able to write an online user review (Haight, Quan-Haase, & Corbett, 2014). Those members' voices will never be captured in the literature unless something is done to address the lack of access or literacy. Even among those that do have access and the requisite skills to write an online user review, there will still be members of the population who will not write a review (Haight et al., 2014). The opinions and experiences of those members will never be captured with this type of analysis.

My skill in these processes is another limitation as this work utilized NLP techniques and qualitative analysis. Others with additional experience in these techniques may obtain different results even following the same methods. Although I was mindful of potential bias during thematic analysis, I ensured that best practices were followed but could not be sure errors or other unconscious biases did not affect this work's results.

Limitations to the Area of Study

This work focused primarily on acute care hospitals in BC. To determine the generalizability of this work nationally or within other provinces, additional study may be required. Population or jurisdictional differences may affect the results. The impact on primary or ambulatory care has also not been determined as both the CPES-IC and user reviews focused on acute care hospitals.

Conclusion

The purpose of this research was to determine if Google free-text user reviews of hospitals in BC contained categories of information found in the CPES-IC, as well as categories of information not found in the CPES-IC. As evidenced by this work's results, categories within user reviews were both within and outside the CPES-IC. With future research, LDA could be used to trend and track categories of patient experience within user reviews that nurses and other health care professionals can use to improve the quality of patient care.

The use of technology-generated data without understanding its intended and unintended effects on health care professionals, patients and the system itself should be avoided. If the goals of health care improvement are to deliver an improved patient experience that is cost-effective and improves population outcomes, we must ensure that well-designed processes and plans for how to use this type of data should be put in place. There is no purpose in implementing technology that will add additional cost and burden without improving outcomes. However, what better way to engage patients in improving patient care than by using their own words to determine which areas of care require improvement.

www.ingramcontent.com/pod-product-compliance
Lightning Source LLC
LaVergne TN
LVHW040907150826
845672LV00007B/1929

* 9 7 8 3 3 8 4 2 6 4 6 1 9 *